EBL

BAI

Deanne Panday is a wellness coac...   .. She uses her
knowledge to conduct workshops, i   ...unal speaker and also
writes blogs on wellness and fitness,   ...ucating people on a holistic
approach to well-being. She was also the fitness expert for Miss India
contestants for eight years. She has written two bestselling books—
I'm Not Stressed and *Shut Up and Train!*.

BALANCE

THE SECRET TO TRUE HEALTH AND HAPPINESS IN 13 WAYS

DEANNE PANDAY

EBURY
PRESS

An imprint of Penguin Random House

EBURY PRESS

USA | Canada | UK | Ireland | Australia
New Zealand | India | South Africa | China

Ebury Press is part of the Penguin Random House group of companies
whose addresses can be found at global.penguinrandomhouse.com

Published by Penguin Random House India Pvt. Ltd
7th Floor, Infinity Tower C, DLF Cyber City,
Gurgaon 122 002, Haryana, India

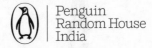

First published in Ebury Press by Penguin Random House India 2020

ISBN 9780143450870

Typeset in Sabon by Manipal Technologies Limited, Manipal
Printed at Manipal Technologies Limited, Manipal

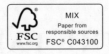

www.penguin.co.in

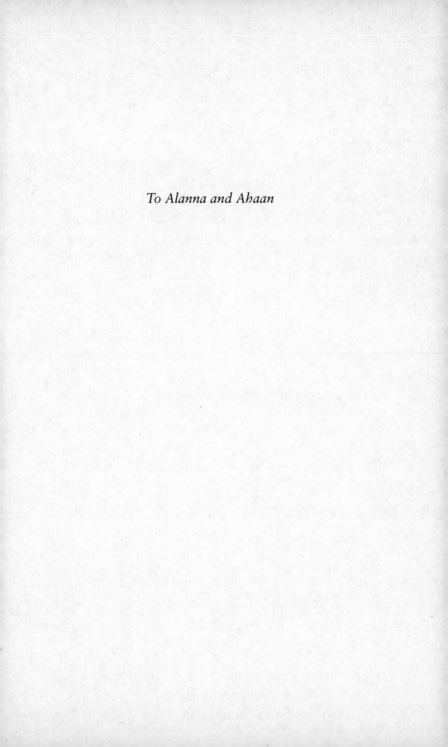

To Alanna and Ahaan

CONTENTS

FOREWORD

I feel lucky to have known Deanne and her family well. While I've known her sister, Alison, for about twelve years, I met Deanne only recently. I have been a model for more than a decade, and Alison is one of India's best choreographers. I've now done more than 500 shows with her. Interestingly, every time I spoke to a model who had become fit really quickly, they credited it to one person—Deanne Panday. Alison herself is very fit, and it isn't just due to genetics. It is because of Deanne.

Deanne Panday has been a well-known fitness guru for some time now. She has trained the most prominent stars in the film industry over the years. Everyone she has trained and partnered with for fitness has been blessed and has achieved great success in their careers. Anyone in the industry who gets to work with Deanne is lucky.

We met for the first time at an award function. Despite all her fame, she has a kind soul and an endearing smile. Even on that first meeting, Deanne complimented me, saying, 'You're the fittest person in the industry.' It takes a lot of confidence and self-assurance to pay someone a compliment like that. You have to be comfortable in your own skin to appreciate others. And that's what stood out to me about Deanne. That is how our friendship began.

To me, Deanne is divinity in a city like Mumbai. The first time I travelled with her, I realized that despite her social life, she is a person who enjoys the simple things in life. She doesn't drink or smoke, but, most importantly, she doesn't talk about others behind their back. She is a ball of positive energy and only revels in the goodness around her. That is what I admire the most about her, and I believe that is what helps her strike a balance between her personal and professional life, between her mind, body and spirit. This reflects in her family life too. Deanne has raised her children so well, shaping them into such confident individuals.

People often ask me about my fitness. When I was three years old, I started playing with swords and sticks. It set me off on my journey to fitness and working out. I was lucky to grow up in an ashram with 800 women and go on to learn kalaripayattu, one of the oldest forms of martial arts in the world. It is believed to have been taught by Lord Shiva to Maharshi Parashuram, who then began the tradition almost 8,000 years ago. 'Kalari' means a battleground and 'payattu' means a playground or a place where one trains for battle. Kalaripayattu was originally derived from animal movements. Every practitioner has to observe and closely follow the movements of one species for a certain amount of time. I have lived with about twenty-five species of animals, watching their movements, trying to experience their emotions and unique instincts—such as the fearlessness of a tiger or the patience of an elephant. *Kalari chikitsa,* or the treatment of battle injuries, is another part of the ancient art form. I have studied both and dedicated my life to martial arts.

My body is my drawing board. It inspires me and challenges me, making me push my boundaries. I treat it as a teacher. Imbibing from nature, cultivating that truth into your being and expressing it through your body is what makes a true and balanced warrior. I have followed these principles and reaped rewards in fitness and in life.

Balance is important in every aspect of life and I am glad that Deanne has written about it in detail in this book. According to kalaripayattu, there are seven systems in our body—muscular, skeletal, respiratory, cardiovascular, lymphatic, visceral and neuromuscular. All of them have to be in sync, and this is what her book *Balance* offers to readers through the circle-of-life programme. Deanne herself practises all that she mentions in the book, and it shows in the loving and kind way she treats her family and friends—just as she would treat herself. Deanne has learnt all this through her own experiences—she is self-taught and self-trained.

When Deanne and I meet, we end up talking only about wellness and our respective spiritual journeys. Her focus is on how to grow as a human being. We've spent hours discussing how to develop ourselves and get better at what we do. I don't meet people such as Deanne often, and I know that her authenticity and positive outlook to life make everyone vie for her time. Deanne's spiritual quotient is as high as her fitness quotient—and it makes her a very balanced person. Most fitness experts focus on the first system—the muscular system—and then the skeletal one. But Deanne looks beyond it. And thus her neuromuscular and lymphatic systems are also perfectly balanced and in sync. She is also very particular about energies and can sense a person's energy when she meets them. Through her positivity and genuine empathy, she lifts you spiritually and emotionally.

Deanne is a great student, and we are kindred souls in this aspect. We are receptive to new information and new practices that can help us get better and learn more. The way she learns is the way I learn—by observing and implementing. For instance, I don't have a regular workout regime—I don't work out at a gym. Instead, I focus on strengthening my ligaments and tendons. We need to take care of all the seven systems in our body.

I love every form of exercise that my body is capable of. To be part of a journey, you first have to embark on it. It is the same with fitness. It's all about hard work and dedication. Discipline isn't about waking up early—it is about keeping the promises you make to yourself. Do the 500 push-ups you said you would. The mind and body are deeply interdependent, so you have to make sure they are in balance. For me, the goal is to make sure that the right side of the brain is in sync with the left side. When I learn something new, I practise it in my head a gazillion times, so that both my mind and my body are ready for it.

Since I do my own stunts in my action films, I find that fear is my best friend. In *Khuda Haafiz*, I jumped from a building. I was scared before performing that stunt. I kept thinking, 'What if I miss it?' But fear is the best thing. It makes me think about all that can go wrong. And then, when I do it, I look back and pat myself on the back for conquering my fear—and that's the biggest high I get in life. And then the fear returns for the next stunt. The mind and the body have to be in balance. My advice to readers is that if you find an exercise or movement difficult—let's say a yoga pose—you should attempt it at least once. And then, with practice and the right guidance, you will be able to do it.

I find that Deanne, besides being a fitness guru, is also one of the best counsellors in Mumbai. I am passionate about healing. It is one of the gifts I have that I feel I should share with others. After my healing sessions, where I help people recover from their injuries, aches and pains through breathing, I often refer them to Deanne for post-recovery therapy. I enjoy working with her, and we work in harmony together. Instead of always offering solutions, she patiently listens to one's problems. To use one's ear chakra so completely is a rarity.

Deanne is the best person to talk about balance in one's life because she lives it herself. She has the strength of an elephant, the alacrity of a tiger, the eyes and the kindness of a deer and the focus of an eagle. I wish her all the luck for her book, and I am sure she will continue to transform many more lives.

Vidyut Jammwal
Actor and martial artiste (kalaripayattu)
Part of top six martial artistes in the world by Looper
Winner of two awards at the Oscars of action,
the 5th Jackie Chan International Action Film Week 2019
Part of 10 People You Don't Want to Mess with
in the World by TheRichest

THE CIRCLE OF LIFE

Are you ready to change your life forever?

When was the last time you let go and had fun? I'm talking about dancing like no one is watching, about sitting on a swing and pushing yourself to go higher and higher—when was the last time you really lived?

I'm sure you did all this and more as a child, but you rarely seem to find time as an adult to be truly free. The excitement and joy we experienced when we were younger—untainted by the responsibilities of adult life and everything it brings in its wake—remain unmatched. As children, we played all the time and found joy in the simple things, but as adults we've forgotten how to. We get so caught up in chasing our goals, moving from one task to another and just being busy that we lose sight of the simple joys of life. We work hard but forget to play.

But it's possible to capture that childhood happiness and bring it back into our lives. But just like you need to be reminded to let go and play a little, you also need to be reminded about *how to play*. That is one of the main reasons I called my gym 'Play' when I started it a few years ago. My first instinct was to call it 'Playground', but I soon realized

I would have to let down the six-year-olds who would come knocking on the door during their playtime.

Play evolved to be a place where people could leave their stress at the door and have fun. I wanted it to be a haven people could escape to, to get away from the hustle and bustle of the city and feel the same peace and joy that they felt so easily in their childhood. When we started out, the building had brick walls. When I stood in the space for the first time, I felt that there was no flow of energy and no sunlight in the space. My mind rebelled against the lack of natural light. So I ensured that two of the walls were built entirely of glass, so clients could work out while looking at nature outside. We then changed the seats of the equipment from boring black to orange, to make the place livelier and give off a fun vibe. This was a rare design for Mumbai. It was also risky, because it was unlike the other gyms of the time—but it really paid off. Play soon came to be known for its fun look and people felt it was a space that they could feel free in. My gym was also different because we were one of the first establishments in the country to use biomechanical equipment. We got HOIST machines, which are designed with a deep understanding of biomechanics. The machines supported the movements of the person exercising, reducing stress on the joints and preventing injuries.

I hoped my clients would be inspired by the surroundings I had created. My three-storey playground had yoga and group-dance classes, an expansive gym, a spa and dedicated nutritionists and physiotherapists. I did my best to make sure there was never a dull moment at Play. It was built for playing, where you could be like a child and have pure, unadulterated fun while also strengthening your body. And this is the time, around 2011, that Random House approached me to write my first book on the innate connection between stress and fitness, which culminated in *I Am Not Stressed*.

However, to be honest, there have been times even I have forgotten to play. I've always been told I have a childlike wonder for things. But there have been times when I have failed to hold on to feelings of curiosity and excitement—feelings that have served me well in good times and tough. Fortunately, I have never been afraid to ask why when life has puzzled me and to seek answers within.

I didn't know it then, but when I look back now, I started on this journey towards seeking balance in my life in the mid-1990s, when I suffered a serious setback in my life. The incidents shook me to my core, and I realized I had to focus more on my inner self. I took a conscious decision to become financially independent and be the best mother I could be to my children. It led me to my successful and fulfilling career in fitness, to a determination to find joy within and to practise the art of self-care. Yoga, spirituality and positivity helped me along the way.

I introspected on what I could do to make my life better. I thought about each part of my life and asked myself what would make me happier. I discovered the Institute of Integrative Nutrition in 2016, and the curriculum really spoke to me. It connected with everything I have been practising in my life for the past twenty-five years now. It gave a name and form to everything I had experienced so far. My circle-of-life tool is inspired from what I learnt at the school when I was studying to be a health coach, and what I have learnt from life. I have modified the circle to what I feel each of us needs to achieve balance. That is how I came to form a list of thirteen aspects that lend balance to my life. I call these aspects my 'vital foods', my first source of energy. These are my non-food sources of nourishment. When they are in alignment, every part of my life provides unadulterated joy. These aspects come together to form what I call the circle of life. The correct balance in each of these is what we all need to fuel and nourish us.

The thirteen aspects are:

1. Relationships
2. Home environment
3. Finances
4. Career
5. Health
6. Physical wellness
7. Spirituality
8. Joy
9. Home-cooked food
10. Creativity
11. Education
12. Social life
13. The impact of climate change on health

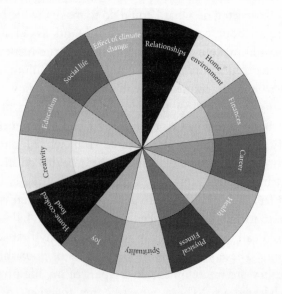

Research shows that good **relationships** help us live longer and deal with stress better.[1] They give us love and our lives meaning. Think about the time a relationship was going through a rocky patch—whether it was with your parents, your spouse, your boyfriend or girlfriend, a sibling, a colleague or a friend. It gave you a lot of angst and stress, didn't it? I'm sure you only felt better when the issue was resolved and the bond went back to normal, or you found a way to accept and understand the issue.

That's how relationships affect us. They make a place for themselves in our heart. We need our relationships to be wonderful for that all-important balance. Striving to make them more fulfilling is a constant battle, and this book will tell you how to have rewarding relationships.

Home is a place that is supposed to make us feel happy, safe and secure. It's the place we return to at the end of a long, tiring day. It's our sanctuary, where we look forward to being the most. Coming home to a welcoming, peaceful and loving family or loved ones is necessary for our emotional well-being, making our **home environment** essential to a balanced life. In the corresponding chapter, I will also talk about how technology can affect family dynamics and how decluttering changes the energy flow of your home for the better.

Similarly, a stable **financial situation** goes a long way in reducing the stress in our lives. For that, we need to work hard, do our best to make smart decisions and understand

---

[1]   L.F. Berkman and S.L. Syme, 'Social Networks, Host Resistance, and Mortality: A Nine-Year Follow-Up Study of Alameda County Residents', National Library of Medicine, 1979, https://pubmed. ncbi.nlm.nih.gov/425958/ (accessed on 25 July 2020).

the importance of money without letting its pursuit take over our lives. And the best way to make money is to have a **career** that you enjoy and are proud of. We spend most of our waking hours at work, so it is non-negotiable that you do it by pursuing what you love and are passionate about. People who love their work are very fortunate, and that's a goal we should all aspire for.

Another aspect that is necessary to create balance in our lives is **health**. It is probably the most important of the thirteen aspects for me and has helped me create balance in the rest of my life. Every night before I go to bed, I pray for the good health of everyone in my life. No matter who you are, what your goal is or what success means to you, one thing holds true for everyone—a healthy body and mind is essential if you want to lead a truly successful and balanced life.

Very few people have spoken about how important gut health is. You cannot be healthy if your gut isn't in optimum shape, no matter how perfect your BMI is or how muscled you are. I can attest to how much it affects every part of my life, from my state of mind to how I look. Without good gut health, you just won't be able to achieve balance.

A large part of your health is determined by **physical wellness**. I love exercising and rarely miss an opportunity to do so. It stabilizes me physically and mentally, and gives me the strength I need to face the world. Along with a healthy body, we all need a healthy mind too. And **spirituality** is the best way to achieve it.

We live in stressful times, and constantly feel like we are being pulled in different directions, leaving us drained and unfulfilled. To ensure we live every day to its fullest, and find happiness in even the most ordinary experiences, we need to be spiritual as well as **joyful** every moment.

For the body and the mind to function the way they should, we need to feed them well. There is no replacement for nutritious **home-cooked food**, using the cleanest ingredients we can find. Food made with love nourishes our body and soul.

Similarly, indulging in **creative activities** is home-cooked food for the brain. In fact, it wouldn't be wrong to call creativity a spa for the brain. Unlock the potential of your imagination and talent, and see how true balance can change your life for the better.

Education is another source of the vital nourishment we need. Learning about the world around us and gaining knowledge is an unmatched source of power. Education impacts our decision-making and critical-thinking skills, and opens up opportunities for us to take on and change our world. My father-in-law once said, 'You can gain knowledge every day till you die', and I try to live by that idea even today. I encourage others to keep learning and educating themselves as well.

A happy **social life** should involve like-minded people who support you in good times and bad. Whether you are an introvert, an extrovert, an ambivert, or just you, an engaging and honest social life will surely enrich your way of living.

An understanding of **climate change** rounds off the circle of life. I don't need to explain why it is important to breathe in clean air. Without an unpolluted environment, it is difficult to live a good life, no matter how happy and fulfilled you are. The only way to ensure that we take care of our environment for ourselves, our children and our grandchildren is to understand climate change and take it seriously. It is integral to our life to connect with nature, to be one with everything. We are all part of the circle of life, each species supporting another in some way, and if this balance is disrupted, life will eventually cease to exist. So every time you abuse this planet, you are abusing a part of you.

We tend to obsess about the food we eat, but to me that is secondary to my 'vital foods', as these form the true circle of life. We should be concentrating on these non-food sources of nourishment, as they make us thrive and provide a deep inner sense of accomplishment and happiness. Unless you understand the importance of vital foods and their impact on your life and health, the food on your plate will add no value to your life. For example, you may have the body you desire by following a strict diet, but if you are struggling to maintain happy relationships with the people in your life, I can assure you that you won't feel fulfilled. Similarly, your life is unlikely to have joy if you're not satisfied with where your career is going. No matter how healthy you are or what diet you follow, you will not thrive if your vital foods are not in balance.

If we don't nourish each area correctly and to the right extent, there will always be a sense of something missing, something you are searching for, and it'll hold you back from leading the best life you can.

It's easy to overlook one or more of the vital foods because of the busy lives we lead today. We tend to get caught up in the daily cycle of life, without any time to introspect.

The thirteen aspects encompass our professional and personal lives. It is only when everything is in sync that we feel whole—the idea that everything that matters is the way it should be, that we are in *balance*.

Finding balance is an ongoing, lifetime project. It is not a fixed goal, at the end of which you will have a calm and peaceful life. Balance is a way of living. Just like anything important and meaningful, you have to work towards achieving it. The pressures of life tend to push us towards imbalance, so it won't be easy to break that cycle, but once you realize the power and peace that comes with balance, you'll never lose sight of it. The role each vital food plays in your life will differ, depending on your circumstances. For example, if your career is an area you face issues in or if it's not possible to switch to something of your choice, you must look to increase the role of spirituality, relationships, joy, creativity and social life to achieve that balance.

The following chapters will tackle each of these aspects in detail and give you simple, workable tips on maintaining balance in your life. The circle of life works on a simple principle. Take a piece of paper and draw the circle on it, divided equally into its thirteen aspects. Take a few minutes to think about each aspect and evaluate its current standing in your life. If you're satisfied and happy with it, place a dot towards the periphery. The more dissatisfied you are with it, the closer it should be to the centre. For instance, if you'd like to be creative but haven't yet found the time for it, place a dot near the centre. If you are thoroughly fulfilled with your career, mark a dot on the outline. Once you're done, join the dots. Ideally, it should form a perfect circle, which tells you there is complete harmony and balance in your life. If you have a perfect circle, you are incredibly lucky. But it's more likely that your circle will look like an amoeba.

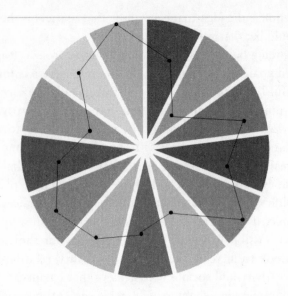

Of course, the aspects that score low are the ones you need to work on. Also, ask yourself a few questions:

- Did an evaluation of some of the vital foods surprise you?
- How do you feel about your life as you look at your circle of life?
- Which of these elements would you most like to improve?
- How do you see yourself go about making these changes?

All of us deserve to thrive in our lives and not just survive. However, the circle is unlikely to always be balanced. We have to constantly work towards achieving that balance, because life throws problems at us every once in a while.

It's like walking a tightrope in a circus. Some acrobats have to walk on a thinner tightrope and some are lucky to start off on a thick one, which makes their journey easier. But regardless of how thick the rope is, it takes true dedication and love for oneself to get to the other side. With enough determination and drive, even the acrobats on the thinnest ropes reach their destination. These are the ones who are remembered the most and who win over the audience.

Our lives have become increasingly complex over the years. Relationships are under strain, our jobs take up most of our days, we have to travel longer hours and our aspirations are so much more. All these take an invisible toll on our minds and bodies. This invisible toll is nothing but stress. It appears when the demands of a particular situation far exceed what we think we can cope with. There are two types of stress. Acute stress is what we experience on a daily basis. These can be dealing with traffic, annoying neighbours, a mean colleague, a thoughtless boss or lack of privacy. Acute stress doesn't linger for a longer period of time. On the other hand, there's chronic stress, which becomes a constant in your life. It could happen because of the death of a loved one, a nagging health issue, a relationship roadblock or financial difficulties. While acute stress can be managed and, in fact, even help you face challenges and perform better, chronic stress can have devastating effects on your body. In the long run, it even affects your body and can manifest as hypothyroidism, obesity, osteoporosis and hypertension. Over time, chronic stress can weaken your immune system as well. It can damage cells in the brain and affect your learning and memory. Chronic stress has a bearing on fertility too, and is known to increase the possibility of miscarriages. In fact, chronic stress has been linked to type 2 diabetes, hypertension, coronary heart disease and cancer.[2]

Stress, at its core, is the body's reaction to harmful situations—whether they're real or perceived. When you feel threatened, a chemical reaction occurs in your body that allows you to act so that you can prevent injury. This reaction is known as 'fight or flight', or the stress response. During a stress response, your heart rate increases, breathing quickens, muscles tighten and blood pressure rises. This is our body's way of saying that it is ready to act. This is how our bodies protect us in stressful situations. However, in this modern generation, because of the imbalance in our circle of life, our body is constantly in fight-or-flight mode. Thanks to the multiple responsibilities we juggle, the body and the mind are rarely at rest. Think of a regular day in your life. You are tired from work the previous day and hence snooze the alarm a few times before you get out of bed. You drink more coffee than required to keep yourself awake. Then you rush to cook for yourself or your family before heading out for work. The traffic on the roads and the crowd in public transport only add to your stress. Once you reach office, work has already piled up, and there are days when your

---

[2]   Frans Pouwer, 'Does Emotional Stress Cause Type 2 Diabetes Mellitus? A Review from the European Depression in Diabetes (EDID) Research Consortium', Center of Research on Psychology in Somatic Diseases (CoRPS), Tilburg University, 2010, http://www.discoverymedicine.com/Frans-Pouwer/2010/02/11/does-emotional-stress-cause-type-2-diabetes-mellitus-a-review-from-the-european-depression-in-diabetes-edid-research-consortium/#:~:text=Results%20of%20longitudinal%20studies%20suggest,life%20events%2C%20and%20work%20stress (accessed on 25 July 2020).

boss is in a bad mood. When the day finally ends, you drag yourself home before repeating the whole routine the next day all over again.

Our nervous systems don't know when to be at ease and when to manage stress. The fight-or-flight response was designed to protect your body in an emergency by preparing you to react quickly. But when the stress response keeps firing all day, it could put your health at serious risk.

The vital foods provided by the circle of life will help you through such moments. It will feed your soul, while the secondary foods feed your body. It has worked wonders for me, and I know it will do the same for you.

The Clean-Your-Life Quiz

I have devised a small quiz so you can attempt to gain better balance in your circle of life. You have to write a yes or a no against the statements below. Only write yes when the statement is always true. Otherwise, say no, even if it's sometimes or usually true. And if you come across a statement that doesn't apply to you, write yes.

- My home is neat and clean.
- My appliances, machinery and equipment work well.
- My clothes are all ironed and clean, and make me look great.
- My bed/bedroom lets me have the best sleep possible.
- I live in a home that I love.
- I have adequate time, space and freedom in my life.
- I rarely eat sugar.

- I rarely watch television.
- My teeth and gums are healthy.
- My cholesterol count is healthy.
- My blood pressure is healthy.
- I am aware of the physical and emotional problems I have, and I am now taking care of all of them.
- I have a fulfilling life beyond work.
- I currently save at least 10 per cent of my income.
- I pay my bills on time.
- My income is stable.
- I know how much I must have to be financially independent, and I have a plan to get there.
- I live well within my means.
- I have sufficient medical insurance.
- I regularly tell my parents that I love them.
- I get along with my siblings.
- I get along with my co-workers.
- I have communicated or attempted to communicate with everyone I've hurt, even if it wasn't fully my fault.
- I have a circle of friends and family who love and appreciate me for who I am more than just what I do for them.
- I have fully forgiven those who have hurt or damaged me, intentionally or otherwise.
- I make requests rather than complain.
- I spend time with people who don't try to change me.

Add up the number of times you said yes. The total will give you an indication of your circle of life. The more 'yes'es you have, the more balanced your circle of life. You can revisit the quiz regularly to see how much your life has changed. As vital foods begin to satisfy you more and more, you will watch your score increase over time. If you have more nos than yeses, this book will guide you to change that and achieve balance.

How This Book Will Help You

I have been living a fitness-focused life for as long as I can remember. I've learnt a few things along the way that have only strengthened my resolve to keep fitness at the forefront of my life. One of them is the sheer, incredible power of the human body.

I have struggled to find a word that fits the wonderful things our bodies are capable of doing, and haven't found a better than this—a biocomputer. The human body is smarter and more intelligent than the best computer in the world. You can push it to limits you didn't think were even possible, and you can make it do whatever you want it to. All it requires is that we take care of it. We need to give our body nourishment—both mental and spiritual, as well as food to sustain it.

Sounds simple enough, doesn't it? It is, but only if you have the facts. There is so much information out there these days, and not all of it is verified. With so much coming at you at the same time, it is understandable that you are confused. That is why the book you're holding in your hands is the definitive guide to striking the right balance in your life and living your best life.

This book is an attempt to improve your health and happiness in every way. The solution to a better life is within us. All we need to do is understand what's wrong when our life isn't where we want it to be. I rarely fall sick, and at the age of fifty-one, I'm the healthiest and fittest I have ever been. I have been able to do that because I put my mental and physical health first. The virtues of self-care aren't popular yet, so I want to reinforce their importance. Self-care isn't selfish; in fact, we should always be available to ourselves. You can begin that by asking yourself what really matters to you. Make a list. Mine includes family, fun, food, sleep, growth, health, love, relationships and connecting to people. I encourage you to take ten minutes from your schedule and make a list for yourself too. Once you've made your list, ask yourself this: What are the things holding me back from ensuring my list is always ticked off? What holds me back is time and knowledge. I sometimes feel I don't have enough information and time to do something new, such as learn a new skill, say, baking bread. The final step towards making life better and more wonderful for yourself is to figure out ways in which you can change.

People don't change in life based on what they know— they change based on how they feel. That is such an important thing to remember when you're seeking any sort of change in your life. Let me illustrate that with an example. We all know someone who smokes, who we wish would give up the habit. We keep chiding them to quit smoking, but they don't listen to any reason we have to give. Pointing out the dreadful effects of smoking on their lives also doesn't help. Why is that? It is because the smoker already knows the ill-effects of the habit. They know it is harmful for them. But they won't give up unless they are ready to do so themselves. It is only when the smoker feels it is time to quit will he or she take that step. Similarly, someone may have the bad habit of always being late, which doesn't affect them physically but could be an indication of some other issue.

We all need to bring about change when we feel it is necessary for us. This book will give you a lot of information on the whys and hows of change, but it is only when you start applying it and feel good about yourself that you can implement the change that you want.

I want you to genuinely enjoy the solutions and the journey towards balance this book offers. Only then will it fulfil my aim of helping you. Otherwise, this will be just another book you'll buy and forget about in a few months. The answers, I promise, won't overwhelm you—they will gently guide you to a place you wish to be. My sincere wish is that the book will set in motion a chain reaction, where you recommend its simple solutions to the people you love and they do the same to the ones in their lives. That way, we will help bring balance to the lives of those we love the most.

MY JOURNEY

She believed she could, so she did.

When I was twelve, all the girls around me were crushing on Rajesh Khanna. I, on the other hand, was busy watching another icon on TV. It was the time when Jane Fonda had introduced the world to home fitness by releasing her range of videocassettes, and my sister and I were hooked. Every day, after school, she and I would pop in the cassette of Jane Fonda's iconic ninety-minute workout video and follow what we saw on TV. In hindsight, that was the beginning of the journey that has brought me where I am today. The kick I got out of the workout made me go back to it every day. Since then, I've tried a lot of different disciplines, and learnt along the way what suits me best. Now, at fifty-one, I am the fittest I have ever been. My body is tougher, my mind stronger and my outlook unassuming and unrestrained.

But that wasn't always the case. I grew up a shy child and was usually the least confident girl in a room. One of my earliest memories is of wearing a Native American outfit for a fancy-dress competition in school and forgetting all the lines I had prepared because I froze on stage. I was also mildly dyslexic, but I didn't know that at the time. I only realized I was a couple of years ago. But it's probably what I can attribute my creativity to, as most people with dyslexia are often highly creative. It encourages me to seek out and express in other forms, and helps me use any particular situation to my advantage.

Four years after discovering Jane Fonda's home workout videos, I was yearning to learn more about fitness. So, when I found a summer job at sixteen, I saved all my money for a gym membership. All those years ago, only five-star hotels had gyms, and they were quite expensive. But I was determined to make my body stronger, and so I signed up. I began lifting weights and enjoyed myself thoroughly. In fact, soon, I was lifting more than the men around me at the gym. It made my boyfriend at the time (and now husband) quite jealous, as I could lift more than him. At that time, I didn't know any other woman who lifted weights.

I also started to learn yoga at the same time. It was an unusual choice, because it was then looked at as an exercise for the elderly. But I am thankful to have learnt the life-changing benefits of meditation and pranayama thirty years ago—way before it gained so much popularity. The combination of gym exercises and yoga held me in good stead when I faced probably the biggest challenge of my life a few years later.

When I was twenty-six, I went through a terrible heartbreak. It left me bewildered, unable to understand how and why something so awful was happening to me. The brain registers emotional pain in the same way it registers physical pain, which is why when we have been hurt beyond imagination, we feel the heartbreak as acutely as physical hurt. That is how it felt to me. I couldn't fathom why I had to endure so much pain. But even amid that foggy state of mind, I knew I was not going to let that define me. I had my family to look after. In such tough moments, we all have two choices: We can either feel sorry for ourselves or change the narrative. I took charge and dove head-first into learning all that I could about fitness. I turned my pain to power.

A few years into my marriage, I had two children and I was a housewife. On the side, I wrote fitness columns for newspapers and magazines. But since I hadn't trained professionally, I felt I needed to know more so I could provide accurate information to my readers. I travelled to Australia for a two-week course. Once there, I realized I had so much to learn that my course wasn't going to be enough. My children were four and two years old then, and I didn't want to be away from them for months. But I also knew that I wouldn't be able to travel to Australia again to study, so I made the tough decision to stay back for four months, learn as much as I could and then come back home to my babies. Those four months changed my life. It was a turning point for me.

A week after I returned to Mumbai, I was offered the prestigious job of training the Miss India contestants. I was so surprised by the offer that I couldn't even give them an answer immediately. I excused myself, went to the restroom, did a small jig and calmly went back and told them I'd be honoured to take up the job. I now had a chance to do what I loved so much.

For me, fitness is another word for self-love. Taking care of my body, and also my mind's needs have given me unparalleled joy over the years. It has also given me the tools to face life's many challenges. One of the best decisions I made at the start of my journey was to listen to my body. It has always given me feedback on whether I have fed it well, if the exercises I did suited it—and even when it needed rest. That one simple choice is why, from the embers of my personal setback, I could become the woman I am today. It is said that you become more beautiful from being broken, and I truly believe that. In fact, I am now thankful for that experience. Had it not happened, I would not have been the strong woman I am today and probably would have had a different life—one where fitness and self-love didn't come to me naturally. During that setback, I had several sleepless nights, wondering how I would ever be happy again. But my career was my salvation. I got out of bed every morning, eager to exercise at the gym.

That phase taught me to be thankful for everything in my life—the good parts and the challenges. I am not romanticizing pain or heartbreak, but I now know that difficult roads lead to beautiful destinations. But only if you have the courage to take the path less traversed.

Looking back, I am proud that I conducted myself with integrity, dignity and grace. The few friends who have been privy to my journey agree with me. The pain of the heartbreak was so severe that I could have reacted badly. But that's just not who I am. I am a private person and deal with my issues quietly. In fact, this is the first time I have publicly spoken about the experience that has played such a large role in shaping my life.

Sometimes, people take the support of alcohol or drugs to navigate tough times, but that's never a good idea. When you go through bad times, you will come out stronger. Alcohol, drugs and prescription pills are not the answer. There is no option but to wake up and face your problems.

There is no doubt that certain substances release chemicals that help ease mental and physical pain. But, in the process, the dependence we develop on the chemicals fail our bodies, minds and hearts—and this is why it isn't worth it.

There are safer, effective, more permanent ways for one to push through hard times. Resorting to a substance is resorting to an altered consciousness, which makes you view the world in a way it is not supposed to be viewed on a daily basis. You are pulling yourself away from the truth, from the pain, but also unknowingly from yourself. But by the time you realize this, more often than not, you're lost in a void that can only be filled by that substance, and every time you resort to it, the void just keeps growing deeper and darker, sucking you in.

My fitness journey not only made me mentally tougher, it is also the reason I have enjoyed good health all these years. I am a bronchial asthma patient—I have been one since I was born. I have patches in my lungs that make it difficult for me to breathe. I would get attacks regularly and have taken medicines for it most of my childhood. But by becoming stronger with my fitness journey and eating what suited my body, I have cured myself of this health issue. I haven't taken any medication for the asthma since I turned sixteen, and haven't had a single attack since then. I don't need to constantly carry an inhaler around either. Thanks to regular exercise and the care I take of my body, I also don't get colds, coughs or even viral fever. So there has never been any real need to take any allopathic medicines. In fact, antibiotics are rarely the answer, unless you are suffering from a major infection. According to a new study conducted by researchers at MIT, the Wyss Institute for Biologically Inspired Engineering, part of Harvard University, and the Broad Institute in the Unites States, 'Drugs are producing changes that are actually counterproductive to the treatment effort. They reduce the bacterial susceptibility to antibiotics, and the drugs themselves reduce the functional benefit of the immune cells.'[1] Sometimes it is necessary to take antibiotics, but too many people turn to them for minor issues that can be resolved without medication.

Years of hard work, good eating habits, yoga, introspection, meditation and fulfilling relationships have helped me achieve perfect balance, and people often ask me how they can have it too. A lot of it is a result of the self-love I turned to all those years ago. It allowed me to tap into an inner calm and peace, and has brought such contentment into my life that petty things do not bother me any more. It has changed me as a person. Now I struggle to understand the need to hanker after material things. I seek the simple joys of life—seeing butterflies flutter, appreciating the colours of flowers, and feeling the sand under my feet rather than buying expensive bags, shoes and phones. When my friends go to Goa to party, I look forward to staying home and doing yoga. While they go shopping when travelling abroad, I would rather go for a walk in the park. While they're at the bar, you'll find me at the beach. I like to play and dance in the rain, and have often been chided by my friends for behaving like a child. But what they forget is that all of these little things have let me find balance in my life. I love the joy that simple things bring and the contentment of good relationships and family life. I enjoy holidays

---

[1] Jason H. Yang et al, 'Antibiotic-Induced Changes to the Host Metabolic Environment Inhibit Drug Efficacy and Alter Immune Function', *Cell Host & Microbe*, 2017, https://www.cell.com/cell-host-microbe/fulltext/S1931-3128(17)30455-9 (accessed on 26 July 2020).

with my daughter. She still loves to shop, but she's young and will someday see the world as I do and find the same contentment that I have. Of late, my son has been learning to play the guitar. Just listening to him play brings me so much joy as well.

This balance has taught me to love being by myself and enjoy my own company. I know so many people who need company for everything they do—whether it is to sleep, shop, travel or, sometimes, to even visit the restroom at a restaurant. Sitting and observing the beauty of nature's bounty and forest-bathing (taking in the atmosphere of the forest through the senses) are some of my favourite things to do. On a recent trip to the Maldives with my friends, they woke up early to spend an hour at the hotel's gym while I sat on the sand and enjoyed the sight of the azure waters. I could not stay indoors when it was so beautiful outside. If it were up to me, the planet would be full of long beaches and lush forests, with a gym at the centre of it all.

This is the person I have been for more than ten years now. I am glad to have found the balance that others seek. There have been times when people haven't understood me. A friend once even asked me if I was from another planet, because I never grumbled about the weather, I was happy with the little joys of life and I tried to see the beauty in everything. I wish I could explain how true happiness makes the little annoyances of life fade away. Some of my friends have found the same balance by choosing the same path I did ten years ago, but there are others who are still more concerned about superficial things.

The joy I have found is within me, and I realize I don't need anyone other than my family, children and close friends. That is why I love spending time on my own. The change has left me unaffected by people who are judgemental. Our vibes and values are so different that I prefer to stay away from everything that is malicious or negative. I make personal growth and development a priority. I celebrate the life I am living because I find beauty in everything. I have always celebrated being different. In the process, I have lost some of my friends, but others who understand me are still a crucial part of my life, and will always be.

Strict No-Nos of My Balanced Life

Over the past decade, I have compiled a list of five things that have had no space in my life over the past few years. They were disturbing the calm I was building around me and threatened to disrupt the peace I wanted to live with. Here's what I compiled:

Gossiping and small talk: Gossiping gives me no joy, because it is always about other people. We can't know everything about the lives of others and why they do the things they do. They have their reasons, none of which we are privy to. So what's the point of talking about things we don't have complete knowledge of? Similarly, small talk goes nowhere and is a waste of energy, and I'd rather talk about something more productive and meaningful than the weather.

Fake and insincere friends: Who needs such people in their lives, anyway? All of us should have well-meaning, loving friends who are there for us in good and bad times. Good friends add indescribable joy and laughter to our lives, and those are the ones we should keep close. At their very core, people don't really change. So you can either let go of them or find a way to deal with them in a way that is least harmful to you.

Violent movies: I don't like the blatant aggression and anger on display in violent movies. Scenes of blood and gore are not my cup of tea.

Meaningless parties: I only attend birthday, anniversary or celebration parties of my friends and family, or if it is an event related to work. I don't attend parties just because I have been invited. I'm particular about being there for my friends and hold those values dear to me. I am not interested in Page 3 parties just to be seen. It makes me uncomfortable. I don't need external validation. What I have and who I am are enough.

Red meat: Red meat, such as pork and beef, have more cholesterol and saturated fat than chicken and fish. It has also been linked to type 2 diabetes. Lean or plant-based proteins put you at a lower mortality risk than a diet rich in red meat. But if you have to have red meat, opt for grass-fed meat and not factory-farmed.

My Diet and Exercise Regimen

Since my work is so public, people often ask me what kind of meals I eat and exercises I follow. I'll answer the easier one first. My physical activity of choice is lifting weights. I lift weights more than I do cardio, simply because I feel they suit me more. But I don't neglect the cardio aspect. I don't run on the treadmill because it is bad for the knees and lower back. Instead, I do a power walk, or use the elliptical, cycle or rowing machine. I also do yoga and meditate every day, both of which have changed my life immeasurably. In the past few months, I have concentrated more on what I do at the gym than on yoga. I wanted to see how much I can push my body to get stronger. I was testing its limits. But that meant I could not do yoga every day. As usual, my body started giving me signals that I needed to get back to it. My mind wasn't as calm as always, so I managed to bring back the balance by fitting yoga into my everyday self-love routine.

As for my meals, I eat a mostly plant-based diet and, sometimes, eggs. I love all vegetables—there isn't one you can name that I don't like. I gave up red meat about eighteen years ago because my sister's friend developed tapeworm from eating pork and almost died. Growing up, pork vindaloo was a dish my mother made regularly, because my family is part Portuguese. I miss the nostalgia of the pork vindaloo, but giving up red meat has made me feel so much better that I never went back. A lot of us grow up with certain habits, but we don't feel the need to break the cycle until something shakes us up. It's okay to let go of things if they are harming you. That's what I have done with some of the food I used to eat when I was younger.

For breakfast, I have two small idlis and two or three seasonal fruits. I also have a small bowl of almonds and walnuts that I soak the night before, and a small cup of tea with lactose-free or almond milk, with a little bit of coconut sugar. I have a small shot of coffee before I leave for the gym. However, I have one or two glasses of water immediately before that, so that the coffee's potency is diluted. I'll explain this is in more detail in the chapter on diets. Through the rest of the day, I have a vegan protein shake, coconut water, lemon water, apple-beetroot-carrot juice and herbal tea. Since the system tends to get acidic over the day, I have made a conscious choice to switch to alkaline water. I keep two bottles of alkaline water aside, which I keep sipping throughout the day. In one I add chia seeds, organic aloe vera pulp and extra-virgin cold-pressed coconut oil. In the other I add a few drops of chlorophyll and some sour lime to give it taste. Lunch is always a home-cooked meal. It includes some protein with lentils and pulses, different kinds of salad, tofu, sweet potato, yam and rice. One of the best tricks I have learnt is to add vegetables to everything I eat, whether it is salads, rice or curries. My dinner is very light—I just have a big glass of green juice and half an avocado.

The green juice has blended crisp lettuce, romaine leaves, butterhead lettuce, Swiss chard, lollo rosso lettuce, red oakleaf lettuce, white pakchoi, baby spinach, red Russian kale and arugula leaves. The healthy concoction gives me a lot of energy. While I use raw vegetables in my juice, I've been told having it this way isn't ideal. However, I have it because it agrees with me. That doesn't mean it will suit everyone, so you should try it a couple of times and see how it affects you before making it a habit. If it does suit you, the green juice has excellent benefits. It requires hardly any digestion, so its nutritional goodness gets into your system rapidly while also giving your digestive system a rest. Additionally, greens have chlorophyll, which oxygenates your body. They also help you lose weight, improve focus, provide mental clarity, improve bone and joint function, build a stronger immune system, and result in healthier hair, skin and nails.

In addition, I also take a turmeric tablet, calcium, spirulina, vitamin B complex, probiotic and an Ayurvedic ashwagandha tablet every day. Eating a diet rich in leafy greens also offers numerous health benefits, such as reduced risk of obesity, heart disease and high blood pressure. I am also mindful of the products I use on my body. My toothpaste is herbal and my skincare products are made of Indian organic ingredients.

A year ago, I got a genetic mapping test done. The results were a wonder. That's when I found out that everything I had been doing regarding my health, fitness and life was correct. All the decisions I had been making—whether it was to go vegetarian or reduce my coffee intake—were exactly what I needed to do. The test showed that coffee was harmful for me. My body had been giving me signals that it wasn't suiting me, because it would leave me anxious, constipated and sometimes even make me shake. According to the test, my body does not absorb B12 vitamins naturally. And since they play an essential role in the production of red blood cells and DNA, as well as the proper functioning of the nervous system, I immediately started having a B12 supplement, and every few months take an injection that is a concoction of B vitamins. The test showed that I had tested negative for smoking addiction, but I could get addicted to alcohol because it was in my genes. Because of my healthy lifestyle, I don't turn to alcohol even for recreational fun.

The choices I have made aren't difficult. You can make similar ones too. I won't recommend mine to you because your body is different. What works for me won't necessarily work for you. All I can recommend is that you do what is needed and best for your body. That's the only way I know you can find complete balance in your life. There are, however, some basic values that will guide you, regardless of your individual physical and emotional make-up.

My Core Values

- Being a source of positive changes.
- Doing what I love and loving what I do.
- Setting an example of self-development and growth.
- Living each day with the freedom to choose what's right for me.
- Supporting those around me in the global shift to better health.
- Embracing learning and new ways to do things.
- Creating balance in all areas of life.
- Simplifying everything.
- Breaking out of harmful cycles.

DIET

Food is fuel, not therapy.

Now that you know how important vital foods are to our mental and physical well-being, let's tackle the most common myth—that diets with restricted calorie intake are the only way to lose weight. This chapter will debunk that myth and tell you why you should obsess less about what's on your plate and more about all the thirteen vital foods I spoke about in the preceding chapters. Brace yourself for the truth and read on.

Why Diets Don't Work

As you're getting ready for work in the morning in front of the mirror, you check out your body. You turn to your right and then to your left. Your smile fades. Those stubborn few kilos refuse to drop. Maybe it's time to listen to your colleague who has a miracle cure—a diet she swears helped her look slim for her wedding. And she did look very pretty that day. So you ask her about it at work and start on it the next day. This one's going to be different, you're sure. Over the next few weeks, you notice a considerable difference in your body's shape. Saying no to your beloved potatoes has been difficult, but so worth it. You're proud of what you've achieved so far. But one day, at an office party, the plate of fries looks so tempting. You eat a few at first. But then it's tough to control yourself and you end up having a lot. And before you knew it, potatoes are back, baby. Soon, the weight is back to where it was and you start feeling hopeless again. You believe that you have failed. A few months pass and your best friend tells you about this new diet. And your eyes light up . . .

This is how the story of every diet goes. It begins with enquiry, moves to action, then elation, and then to surrender and finally hopelessness before the cycle begins again. 'Diet' is one of the most abused words today. By definition, a diet is the different kinds of food that a person, animal or community habitually eats. But the way we have come to use the word is a temporary and highly restrictive programme of eating so as to lose weight. Take a moment and list all the diets you've heard of and how they all promised quick weight loss. I can think of Atkins, GM, paleo and ketogenic off the top of my head. Sure, all of these have delivered the desired results, but they have also confused a lot of people, resulting in the diet being misused. That is why when you've completed your diet, you simply boomerang to the unhealthy eating patterns that caused you to gain weight in the first place.

Also, according to some estimates, about 80 per cent of people who lose weight by dieting are bound to regain it in one to five years.[1] Since dieting is a temporary food plan, it won't work in the long run.

---

[1] Brenda Goodman, 'How Your Appetite Can Sabotage Weight Loss', WebMD, 14 October 2016, https://www.webmd.com/diet/

What you need instead is to stop misusing the word 'diet' and begin eating in a balanced manner, one that is tailor-made for you. There's no one diet or weight-loss plan for everyone. All of us are trying to emulate other people. When we learn that certain diets helped our neighbour, a gym friend or an actress, we start following them too. Since all of them are losing weight, they must work. But we are all different. Nutrition should be based on individuals, not on theories. However scientific the diet is, it has to be based on you and what your body needs. All diets are not built for you, your life and your goals.

Instead, they are based on your age, race, gender, culture and activity levels. Let me explain. Our bodies are always changing. The nutrition you need now is different from what you required in the past and will not be the same in the future either. As we age, we tend to burn fewer calories and, therefore, usually need to eat a little less. The changes we go through as we grow older—such as slowing metabolism, diminishing muscle mass, thinning organ tissue and decreasing bone density—means we need different foods and nutrients as we grow older. Simply put, what our body needs at the age of twenty-five is different from what it needs ten years later. So how can the same diet work for different people of different ages?

Similarly, people of different races don't always require the same amount of each nutrient. For instance, type 2 diabetes is more common in India than any other country in the world. Asian Indians are different in the way their cells convert food to available energy, when compared to other

news/20161014/how-your-appetite-can-sabotage-weight-loss#1 (accessed on 27 July 2020).

races. It's quite silly to not have a diet that caters to your racial profile.

There's an Italian woman who works at a spa I visit. She's been working in India for a few years now. She was unwell some time back and most of her clients told her to eat khichdi to feel better. We all know that khichdi is the first line of defence in any illness in an Indian home. She did take up that advice, but this is what she told me: 'Comfort food for me is pasta, because that is what I have grown up with. Khichdi just does not have the same effect on me.' I agree with her, because while khichdi conjures up images of home, well-being and comfort for Indians, it just doesn't mean the same thing to an Italian.

Our genetics also play a significant part in the kind of nutrients our body needs. Some diseases are hereditary and you may be at higher risk of contracting certain illnesses, such as heart disease and diabetes. My husband, for example, has diabetes—there is a history of the condition in his family, including his father. So he needs a food plan that is different from his brother, who doesn't have diabetes.

Culture, too, cannot be ignored when choosing the correct meal plan. For instance, Gujaratis tend to veer towards sweet stuff, while those from Kerala like coconut and rice to be part of the meals they cook. Bengalis, on the other hand, are known to love fish. So if they are suggested an eating programme where they have to give up something that's such an integral part of their culture, the diet is unlikely to succeed.

People eat differently on weekdays and weekends as well. They tend to be stricter with their meals on weekdays and indulge on weekends, when they socialize more.

Men and women, too, eat differently. Because men generally have larger bodies—both height- and weight-wise—and greater muscle mass, they have increased caloric needs, as compared to women. I know someone who is fit and has a big bowl of chicken or mutton keema for breakfast every day. You may baulk at it, but that heavy breakfast suits him.

We eat different foods during different seasons as well. Seasonal produce has twice as much flavour, that extra crunch and an extremely high serving of vitamins, minerals and other essential nutrients. Consuming foods that are not in season may come with a risk of chemicals and preservatives that are applied to fruits and veggies to keep them fresh. Seasonal eating is also usually better for the environment, because foods grown locally require less energy and resources to produce and transport. Winter is the time for warm foods such as soups, with spices to complement them. Hot summers should take you towards cooling foods such as cucumber and watermelon. Monsoon is a time when germs and bacteria thrive in unhygienic conditions, and the high humidity can make our digestive systems sluggish. Thus, eating the right kind of food—such as khichdi with ghee, or bone broths—and taking care of your health becomes important to prevent yourself from falling ill.

In fact, in most cases, it is how your gut reacts to the food you eat that determines your diet. Research has shown that obese people have a less diverse microbiome than thin people, supporting the theory that a variety of healthy gut bacteria are key to health and weight maintenance.

So take a moment and think about it—how can the same diet work for everyone when everyone's gut is built differently?

A Different Diet for Each Person

When Shah Rukh Khan wrote the foreword to my previous book, he told me something I still remember: 'Your workouts are as individual as your fingerprint.' Taking that thought further, I'd like to add that your eating patterns, food choices and diet, too, are just as unique.

These are just some of the reasons that illustrate why one diet does not fit all. Diets focused only on calorie restriction don't guarantee better health. As a health coach, I respect the individual more than the theory. Every diet theory, at some point, will fail. For example, if you start a diet for a couple of months and fall off the wagon, I will blame the diet and not the person. Every time you have been unable to follow a diet, I am sure you believe that you have failed. In fact, it's the diet that has failed. This failure will make you chase another diet and, when that doesn't work, you will look for a new one. You then switch to a new dietician and new workout regimen, which, more often than not, will harm you. This is the beginning of a vicious cycle. I have had to send some of my clients to psychologists because all their efforts to lose or maintain weight have failed and they are unable to cope with it. Yo-yo dieting has also been linked to heart disease, insulin resistance, higher blood pressure, inflammation and, ironically, long-term weight gain.[2] It also affects self-esteem and leads you to doubt your abilities.

---

[2] Eun-Jung Rhee, 'Weight Cycling and Its Cardiometabolic Impact', *Journal of Obesity and Metabolic Syndrome*, 2017, https://www.ncbi.nlm.nih.gov/pmc/articles/PMC6489475/ (accessed on 27 July 2020).

To know what kind of nutrition is right for you, you have to listen to your body. Really listen. Be attuned to it and pay attention to what it is telling you, no matter how subtle it is. I can attest to this because it is by listening to my body that I cured myself of a severe bout of acidity.

About ten years ago, when I was forty-one, I suddenly developed acidity. It shocked me, because I was a healthy person and hardly fell ill. So why was it happening to me? Was age catching up? Was I eating something that was causing this discomfort? When I told my friends about it, I got many recommendations—to try aloe vera, ajwain, apple cider vinegar and allopathic medicines. Everyone suddenly had a remedy at hand. But I wasn't convinced to try these suggestions, as I wasn't sure they would suit me. What's good for one person may not be the same for another. I did, however, take some acidity pills my husband gave me. While those helped for a while, the acidity came back as soon as I stopped the medicines. The tablet was only suppressing the problem and not addressing it. It was time to take charge.

I decided to conduct an experiment, at the end of which I hoped to figure out what was wrong. The first step I took was checking the kitchen cabinets. Everyone at home was shocked, because I can't cook and rarely go into the kitchen unless I have to supervise something. Once everyone's jaws had lifted off the floor, I realized that my kitchen was full of packaged and processed masalas. It was all so different from my grandmother's kitchen, where she used to grind all the spices herself and store them in bottles and not in plastic packets. When did I go the packet-masala way? I immediately made sure that our cook, who has been with our family since she came to Mumbai twenty-five years ago, would use only freshly ground masalas from now on. I left her with instructions to prepare the masalas the way she would in her village. That was the first change I made.

Step 2 was reducing my coffee intake. I know that coffee is known to cause acidity and my three–four cups every day weren't helping. I used to have two cups before exercising in the morning and the remaining two later in the day. I had noticed that the coffee would sometimes make me anxious and hyper, but since I loved it, I had ignored these signs. I reduced my consumption to just one coffee shot before the gym and also began to dilute its effect by having a couple of glasses of water beforehand.

Step 3 was alcohol. I drink only on special occasions— that, too, just one or two glasses of wine. I knew that alcohol didn't suit me, because, at the end of the second glass, I would feel weird and it just wouldn't sit well. I hadn't yet done anything about that, but it was time to get serious. I cut out alcohol completely.

Soon, my acidity had reduced considerably. But it still didn't go away. The next course of action was to change my eating habits with regard to milk and wheat, both of which are known to cause acid reflux. Milk would leave me feeling bloated, so I decided to switch to lactose-free milk to see if it suited me. I began to feel much better. I haven't had a test to know if I am lactose-intolerant, but I know this milk suits me. Next, I turned to evaluating the wheat in my diet. I gave up white bread, but substituted it with sourdough.

The final step in my journey to curing acidity was the elimination of my favourite snack—popcorn. Popcorn feels like a light and healthy snack, but it's actually very carb-dense. Some popcorn also has trans fat added for a longer shelf life. This, too, can upset digestion. Within a couple of months, I knew I had said goodbye to acidity for good. It has never been back since, even when I sneak in the occasional bowl of popcorn. Even if I do have some of the food that caused acidity, it doesn't affect me, because I cleansed my body thoroughly at that time. I healed myself on my own and at my own pace. The elimination diet worked because I listened to my body. It was giving me signals whenever I fed it food that it rejected, and made the necessary changes. There were definitely moments when I was tempted to take an anti-acidity pill, but I stayed the course, remained patient and healed my body. I have not had acidity for years now.

You can begin listening to your body by noting down your mealtimes, what you've eaten and how much. Now comes the slightly tedious part. Observe how you feel immediately after eating, then two to four hours after eating, and the next day as well. Write down what you feel. At the end of a week, you will be able to answer these questions: How did you sleep? How were your energy levels? What changes did you notice in your mood and behaviour? Did any of your food choices manifest in how you felt?

This is how you will know what signals your body is sending you. I understand this may sound boring, but I haven't found a better way of listening to my body than maintaining a diary. It takes a lot of disciple to do this, but that's the least you can do for your body. That's how I got rid of my acidity, and I know it can help you benefit too. You don't always need an expert to tell you what you need. Your body is enough, only if you pay attention.

Cut Out the Complex

Everybody's got an opinion on nutrition. Whether it is solicited or not, you will have people giving you advice on the right foods to eat. One of the reasons nutrition is a tough nut to crack is that because we all eat a variety of food, it's hard for researchers to gauge the body's response to any specific food. With all the information that is directed towards us, we tend to complicate things. Keeping it simple always makes a difference. The clarity that it brings makes life easier to navigate.

The best foundation to creating your own diet plan is to have simple, home-cooked food, and as many fruits and vegetables you can pack into it.

Diets tend to restrict you from eating certain food groups. Either you're told to cut out carbs or fat from your diet. Some only tell you to eat protein and others ask you to cut out rice. The body doesn't react well when it is deprived of a particular food group. If you cut out carbs completely, your body will eventually go into a state of ketosis, where small fragments of carbon called ketones are released into the blood because the body is burning fat instead of carbohydrates. Keto diets might sound appealing at first, but fat is a slower source of fuel than glucose, which means it takes longer for your body to access it, so it will be harder to get going during exercise and other activities. Cutting out carbs altogether can result in fatigue, weakness, dizziness, headaches, irritability and nausea, which can last a few days, or even weeks. Such symptoms are common enough for a term to have been coined to describe the condition—low-carb flu. And not all carbs are bad. Lentils, beans and whole grains are all sources of carbs, but they are usually good for health.

At the same time, fat is also extremely important. It provides energy in a very concentrated format. One gram of fat has nine calories, compared to proteins and carbohydrates, which have four calories per gram. Body fat can also help protect organs and hold them in position. Fats make up the membrane that surrounds every type of cell in the body, and without it, the cell won't function properly.

It's easy to design a plan where people stop eating certain foods, but we all know how tough it is to follow that. There is no reason why you should be food-celibate. Food groups don't need to be given a bad name unless it is sugar, of course, which deserves that moniker.

I have a 9:1 or 4:1 ratio of healthy-to-unhealthy foods I eat every day. I don't believe in depriving myself of food that I love when I want it. And unlike many others, I don't keep track of my calorie intake. Instead, I make sure my food is always nutrient-dense and full of colour. Carrots, beetroot, greens—my meals have all this and more. There is no vegetable I don't eat—I love all of them. I eat my favourite foods, but with healthy options. When I feel like having pizza, I opt for thin-crust pizza and ask for lots of vegetables as toppings. When it comes to rice, I choose a fat grain and throw away all the starchy water. That way, I can eat whatever I want. I don't believe in cheat meals and cheat days. It is better to have smaller amounts of food you crave than restricting yourself to such an extent that you go crazy and eat lots in one day. Abstaining and starving yourself is not good. You have to have a relaxed attitude towards eating food, so don't feel guilty about indulging. Eating food we love is one of the best joys of life. Don't deny yourself that.

Is there an ideal ratio of protein–fat–carbs in the diet? Not really. Grass-fed red meat once a month, organic eggs a couple of times a week, chicken once a week, along with lots of fruits and vegetables, whole grains and legumes is a good mix.

Abstaining is why most people gain weight when they stop dieting. The weight comes right back when you return to your normal eating pattern. The weight appears to come back so quickly because, when you are at your lightest, you tend to gain more weight each day. The lighter you are, the fewer calories you need. If you only need 1,500 calories per day and you're eating 2,000, you're going to gain weight faster than if you need 1,800 and you're eating 2,000. There are only two ways to keep the weight off:

1) Change your overall eating pattern so that you take in, on average, fewer calories than before you went on diet.
2) Start exercising so that you burn the extra calories you take in.

Eliminating food groups, however, is not the silliest diet theory I have heard. There's a baby-food diet, where you eat the way a baby does. It involves replacing one or two meals or snacks a day with baby food—jars of which range in calories from about 20 to 100. Then there's the Second World War ration diet, based on the skimpy rations people had to make do with during the Second World War. Someone told me about the P diet recently, where you stop eating foods that begin with 'p'—potatoes, peas, paneer, etc. I'd like to say a lot about these ridiculous diets, but that would require another book.

What diets do is create a fear of certain foods. Blanket statements that claim that all kinds of rice and potatoes are bad are dangerous. It's best not to put such ideas in your head. The body can determine for itself what is right and wrong for it. All I recommend is that you keep it uncomplicated. Eat fruits and vegetables that have been grown, ideally, in organic soil, and try to go for non-GMO (genetically modified organism) versions. Try to add vegetables to everything you eat. My dal, rice and salad every day include vegetables that go well with them. I use different combinations of veggies so I don't get bored. It's necessary to eat only local produce. We don't know how long ago imported food was harvested and whether chemicals were used to keep them looking fresh and increase their shelf life. Someone recently offered me blueberries from Chile, and I felt my head automatically reject the offer the minute I heard Chile. Food that takes a long time to reach your plate is not the best option, so it's wise to stay away. Don't get carried away by exotic fruits—it is better to eat seasonal and local.

A complex diet, where you have to weigh your food, and count your macros and calories, is useless. It's not possible to do this every day and retain your sanity. You'll be able to do it initially, but eventually it'll start to be a bother, and you'll want to give up. Eating and staying fit is a lot about being at ease with your body and your food, and doing what comes naturally to you.

The Plate Method

I like to use the plate method to organize my meals. It's a healthy way to choose what to eat. It is a conceptual plate that shows the proportions in which various nutrients should be included in every meal.

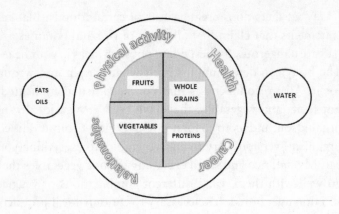

This is what an ideal plate of food should look like—with vital foods as well as secondary foods on it. While one nourishes the soul, the other the body.

I want you to undertake a small exercise. Looking at this plate, fill in the empty plate below with what a typical meal looks like for you.

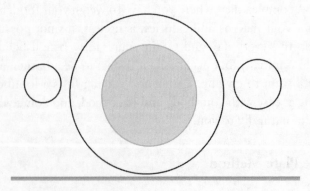

Now compare the ideal plate with yours, mark the difference and answer a few questions.

- How closely does your current diet and lifestyle reflect the ideal plate? What similarities do you notice? What differences do you notice?
- How will you customize your plate to meet your dietary needs?
- How can you create more balance on your plate?
- Are you excited or nervous about making dietary and lifestyle changes?

These answers will help you make better food choices henceforth.

Food Should Feed Your Soul

Health is defined as a state of overall wellness. All everyone talks about these days is going to the gym and what diet they are trying at the moment. But I am sure they would talk about other things as well if they knew that self-care was a journey, not a destination. So many people take care of their bodies and health only when they are getting married, or for a bikini body during a holiday, or after a break-up to show the other person what they're missing. But why not do that every day? Won't life be better that way? Commit to self-love because it is the best sort of prevention against illness. Good health shouldn't be about vanity—it should make you happy. Invest in your body's needs like you would take care of your own child.

I'd like you to take a few minutes and answer the following questions as best you can.

- What does health mean to you?
- How has your idea of health evolved over time?

- Do you dedicate enough time to taking care of your health?
- Do you listen to your body's needs and take action to meet them?

The answers will automatically tell you if you invest enough of yourself in self-care.

A lot of people eat without thinking, and the food they consume doesn't do the job it is supposed to—nourish the body. Our relationship with food is an intimate one, one we cannot afford to mess up. Food is one of our first experiences of being loved, feeling safe and cared for. It is what gives us life and helps us grow. Somewhere along the way, our relationship with food takes a wrong turn and we start defining ourselves as good or bad based on the food we eat. It's common to hear 'Today I was good and I didn't have any sugar at all' or 'I didn't do so well today—I had maida'. It may not seem like a big deal, but the words we use can impact how we feel about ourselves for eating or even wanting to eat certain foods. We tend to impose these labels on our self-worth, which leads to feelings of guilt and shame. It is unhealthy for our physical and mental health to use this language, and can even play a role in developing eating disorders.

You can get over such feelings of guilt and shame by using the food journal we discussed earlier. I don't mean the journal to be a food log for you to track calories or different macronutrients. Instead, write down what you ate and how it made you feel. So if you had a paratha and mixed vegetables for dinner, write down how your body felt after eating it, and what went through your mind before, during and after eating. When you write down your thoughts, you're able to see what you're telling yourself about your food, which I sincerely hope isn't negative. If it is, this should help you slowly turn them into positive sentiments.

For example, if you're having creamy pasta, which isn't technically healthy food, instead of thinking that it's going to make you gain weight, focus on the satisfaction it gives you and how it has lots of carbohydrates to power you through the next few hours.

The most important thing I want you to remember is that when you feed your body quality food, it makes you a healthier person—it doesn't make you a good person. Similarly, when you give it bad food, you are just making unhealthier choices. But that still doesn't make you a bad person. The food is good or bad, not you. Just strive to make healthier choices and you'll do fine.

Cravings

Just as guilt related to food is psychological, so also are most reasons associated with cravings. A client who attended one of my workshops described her craving for her favourite unhealthy food like this: 'Once the thought of what I want to eat enters my mind, it just doesn't leave. I try to distract myself, but every few minutes I go back to that food and how I need just a small bite to satisfy my craving. I can almost taste it in my mouth, and I feel my heart won't settle down until I have had that food.'

This is a pretty good description of how a food craving works. And it's normal. Eating food we love triggers the pleasure centres of our brain, and once you have catered to it, the centre wants to feel that good again. That is why we keep eating the food we love, despite knowing it is unhealthy for us. To control the craving, we have to understand why that feeling occurs in the first place.

Lack of nutrients: If the body doesn't have enough nutrients, it might lead to odd cravings. That is why if you eat healthy, your body knows it has everything it needs to sustain itself and doesn't crave unhealthy food.

Dehydration: We often confuse thirst for hunger and eat something that's not good for us, when, in fact, we should just be drinking some water. The level of our hydration affects our body's electrolyte balance. When we sweat and lose water, we also lose electrolytes such as sodium. This may lead to us seeking out sodium-rich foods after a workout.

Nostalgia: A friend of mine loved to eat cotton candy as a child, so she often finds herself eating the sugar-laden snack when she misses the carefree days of childhood or when she meets up with her school friends. Cravings often come from foods from your childhood. When you feel like this, you may really be seeking the feeling of comfort those foods provided when you were younger.

Yin-yang imbalance: According to traditional Chinese medicine, certain foods are more yin (expansive), while others are more yang (contractive). Within this theory, foods that are too yin or too yang may lead to your craving the opposite in an attempt to maintain balance. You should eat foods that are more neutral (such as whole grains, fruits, vegetables and beans) and avoid those that are extreme, which may lead to cravings. For instance, eating a diet rich in sugar (yin) may cause a craving for meat (yang), or eating too many raw foods (yin) may cause cravings for deep-fried food (yang).

Hormones: When women menstruate, are pregnant or going through menopause, fluctuating testosterone and oestrogen levels can lead to cravings. Stress also alters hormones, which can lead to cravings.

Habit: Sometimes we desire a food or a snack because we're used to having it at a certain time or place. For instance, it's common to feel a drop in energy in the late afternoons and reach for sugary snacks or drinks. Eventually, you start craving snacks during this time simply out of habit.

Foods that are designed to be craved: Yes, and these are called highly palatable foods. A perfect example is sugar. Research has shown that the more sugar people consume, the more they like it. People tend to build a tolerance for sugar and seek it out to create the same pleasurable eating experience that it originally produced. Processed food works in a similar fashion. Processed food affects our metabolism negatively. Over time, it makes us more prone to becoming overweight.

Lack of vital foods: Many people try to cope with debilitating emotions or situations—such as dissatisfaction with a relationship, boredom, stress, lack of inspiration in a job or lack of spiritual practice—by seeking balance through food. Food can provide temporary relief from the discomfort you are experiencing, but using secondary foods to try to fulfil aspects that only vital foods can provide will never be enough. The way to keep a craving in check is to be aware of how exactly you are feeling. First, have some water. Maybe you won't want food after you've hydrated yourself. If the feeling continues, take a moment to tune in to your body. By being mindful and aware, you will be able to distinguish between craving something out of habit and doing so due to actual hunger. And, of course, get your vital foods in order. Listen to what your body is telling you and check if there is a deeper meaning to the craving. That way, you will know if you are craving a particular food or another source of nourishment. I will help you delve deeper into each type of vital food in this book.

How to Manage Your Cravings

Ideally, everyone will eat what's necessary for them. But we are all human and it is all right to indulge once in a while. Having said that, managing the need to binge is important too. While some people feel the urge to eat salty food, others want food laden with sugar. Here's how to manage them.

a. *Salty food*

- When you're cooking at home, use herbs and spices—basil, oregano, cumin, rosemary, thyme, cinnamon, ginger and nutmeg—and a hint of lemon, instead of salt, to add flavour.
- Adding raw garlic to your food gives it a pungent taste. You can even roast it for a sweet and nutty flavour. Similarly, cayenne pepper in any form—fresh, dried or as a powder—packs a spicy, flavourful punch if you want to cut down on sodium.

- Balsamic vinegar comes in many flavours, such as lemon, espresso, cherry, chocolate, apple and garlic, and can be added to many foods.
- While salt does go well with pepper, just pepper on its own brings plenty of flavour to food, usually enough for you to not miss salt at all.
- Cooking with red wine once in a while is also a good alternative to salt.
- Mustard, ketchup and packaged sauces all contain plenty of sodium, as do pickles and papad. Try to replace these with a few slices of tomato instead.
- Vinegar added in small amounts enhances the feeling of saltiness in food without affecting the taste.
- Packaged foods often contain other sources of sodium, such as monosodium glutamate (MSG), baking soda, baking powder, disodium phosphate, sodium alginate and sodium nitrate. Look out for these and stay away from them.

b. *Sweet food*

- Fruits are full of sugar, and they will satiate your sugar cravings easily, along with providing fibre.
- Eat regularly. A longer wait between meals can make you reach for something sugary instead, as your blood sugar might have dropped.
- If you must have sugar, turn to healthier options. For example, opt for darker chocolate, one that has over 70 per cent cocoa.
- There are several vegetables that can do an excellent job of satiating your sweet cravings,

such as beets, carrots, corn, sweet potato, yams and turnips. You can steam, roast and stir-fry them, and season them as you wish with pink Himalayan salt or rock salt and spices.

- You can cook desserts with healthier sugar options, such as maple syrup, stevia, coconut sugar and honey. But remember, what you make is still a dessert, so have a smaller portion of it.

Fighting Cravings with Mindfulness

First, begin by acknowledging that you are craving a particular food. By ignoring it, you will only crave it more. Remember yourself as a teenager. When your parents told you to come back home by a certain hour, you wanted to do the opposite, didn't you? That's what happens when you deny yourself something. The lure of labelling some foods as 'forbidden' leaves you with less control around them.

What Bad Food Does to the Body

One of the most commonly craved foods is the fried snack samosa. Let's see what two different snacks do to our bodies—the ubiquitous samosa and a portion of fruit. Samosa has maida, which has no health benefits whatsoever. Consumption of excess maida can lead to metabolic issues, blood sugar issues, weight gain and heart problems. It is common for maida to be bleached with chemicals such as azodicarbonamide, chlorine gas and benzoyl peroxide. These bleaching chemicals harm the pancreas, affecting its ability to produce insulin. In fact, they are used for inducing diabetes in rodents for laboratory testing. Samosas are re-fried several times so they are hot and appetizing to customers. When food is deep-fried, it leads to the generation of trans fat, which is cancerous in nature. Ever wondered why samosas fill you up so much? Because not only does the dough contain salt, but so does the potato filling. If you're ingesting excess salt, there are high chances of you getting water retention, leaky eyes, poor sleep and dull skin.

I have a few more reasons why fried snacks are so unhealthy for you. But I think I have scared you enough. Now let's see what happens when you snack on fruit when you're hungry. All fruits are a good source of vitamins and minerals. Potassium in fruits reduces the risk of developing kidney stones and helps decrease bone loss as you age. Folate, which is folic acid, helps the body form red blood cells. All fruits have antioxidants that combat free radicals. Fruits are also high in fibre, which helps ward off fats and cholesterol from the body and aid digestion.

Food affects your mood, skin, hair, weight, energy and emotions—basically everything about you. It plays an important role in determining the balance of your life. Have you ever wondered why you tend to eat more when you're feeling low? And why you never crave a salad or healthier food when you do? We have all been guilty of drinking and partying to forget bad incidents and harming our bodies by consuming excess food that isn't good for us. In such cases, what we actually want is love, not the food that we are eating. Fill that void with real emotions and not food. You will physically and mentally feel much better.

A large part of wanting unhealthy food is to do with the brain. Areas of the brain responsible for memory and sensing pleasure are partially to blame for creating those food cravings and sustaining them. Three regions of the brain—the hippocampus, the insula and the caudate—

are activated when you crave a particular food. The memory areas of the brain are responsible for associating a specific food with a reward, and light up when you think of that food item or see a picture of it.

Good, healthy food makes you happy. The hormone serotonin is a chemical messenger that acts as a mood stabilizer. It helps produce healthy sleeping patterns and boosts your mood. Studies show that serotonin levels can have an effect on mood and behaviour, and the chemical is commonly linked to feeling good and living longer.[3] It also helps with sleep, eating patterns, digestion and bowel movement. When you feed your body good food, the levels of serotonin spike, leaving you happier.

Seeking Balance

Emotional eating is almost always unhealthy eating. Rather than expressing emotions and asking for what we truly want, we tend to stuff them down with food, which our bodies translate as comfort and fulfilment. The truth is that the more readily we address emotions, the more healthy our bodies, hearts and minds are. Scientific research has shown that when people have difficulty identifying their emotions and dealing with them, they are more prone to engaging in binge-eating.[4]

---

[3] Simon N. Young and Marco Leyton, 'The Role of Serotonin in Human Mood and Social Interaction. Insight from Altered Tryptophan Levels', *Pharmacology Biochemistry and Behavior*, 2002, https://www.sciencedirect.com/science/article/pii/ S0091305701006700?via%3Dihub (accessed on 27 July 2020).

[4] Alexandra E. Dingemans, Unna N. Danner and Melisssa Parks, 'Emotion Regulation in Binge Eating Disorder: A Review', *Nutrients*, 2017,

When the vital food we need isn't there, we turn to secondary foods to find meaning in our lives. Therefore, the key is to knowing what you feel. Understand the connection between your mood and the food you eat. By deciphering the real meaning behind your cravings, you can get an insight into what's gnawing at you from within. Cravings are a sign that something is off balance or that we need to pay attention to something in our lives.

Your diet is not only about what you eat. It is what you watch, what you listen to and the people you spend time with. Be mindful of the things you put into your body—emotionally, spiritually and physically. We merge our mental, physical, spiritual, sexual and emotional selves together to feed ourselves in a balanced way. That's the best way I know to create health and happiness. You could be the healthiest and fittest person when it comes to food and exercise, but if your vital foods are imbalanced, you can tell that you aren't happy. A happy life is like a big puzzle and all the thirteen vital foods, including secondary food, have to come together to create a balanced life.

Final Thoughts

I want you, dear reader, to take a pledge. Once you promise to follow these steps, I know you will have a much happier relationship with food.

---

https://www.researchgate.net/publication/321232173_Emotion_Regulation_in_Binge_Eating_Disorder_A_Review (accessed on 27 July 2020).

- Eat when you are feeling slightly hungry, not when you are famished.
- Sit and eat in a calm environment with people you love around you. Keep the TV off and your cell phone in another room when you have meals.
- Eat what your body wants.
- Eat until you are satisfied and not stuffed. Excess energy in the body turns into fat, which sticks in and on our organs and disrupts our endocrine system. No matter how healthy our food is, if we eat excess of it and are sedentary, it will be stored as fat.
- Enjoy what you eat. Chew every bite properly. It makes you feel fuller faster and helps in digestion.

And, finally, remember that happiness is an inside job.

How to Stick to a Healthy, Nutritious Plan

Yes, this whole chapter is about why diets don't work. And I sincerely wish that none of you ever starts one. But if you have started one that is suiting you, making you feel better and something you feel that you can make a part of your lifestyle, here are a few tips to help you stay the course.

- Stop thinking of certain foods as bad. It only promotes restriction of those foods, which can lead to unhealthy eating behaviour.
- When you tell yourself something is off-limits, you're likely to think about it more often. So when you do

eventually eat that plate of French fries after having stayed away for months, you're likely to binge on them. That is a natural reaction to depriving yourself of that food.

- Give yourself permission to eat what you want, when you want it. Once you change your mindset, you're less likely to overeat, because you know you can have that food any time. This way, there are no punishments or penalties for straying from the diet and you can always eat the foods you love.

- Eat what you want and not what others do. If you've gone out with friends and others want to share a plate of nachos while you'd prefer sautéed vegetables, order for yourself and not the table.

- Don't punish yourself with a workout if you're going to eat something indulgent that day. Similarly, working out more than required because you went out partying the night before isn't good either.

Why I Love Eating Alone

I spend quite some part of my day alone. I do the things I want at such times. I read up on my work, so I can offer the best to my clients, I play with our pet dog, Peach, and I exercise or watch a show or movie my friends have recommended. I love spending time with myself, because it leaves me calmer and with more clarity. I spend a large part of that time with myself in silence.

I also visit detox retreats on my own. I don't miss company at all because my focus is on making myself healthier. While the retreats have a common dining room, a lot of them have single tables so people can eat alone. 'Silence' is written in a large font in the room, because eating quietly on your own has wonderful benefits. I am able to give the food I am eating my complete attention, without the distraction of phones or people. That way I don't gulp down the food and, instead, chew it well. I am also more attuned to the taste and smell of the food I'm eating, which makes a meal a much more enjoyable experience.

RELATIONSHIPS

Only you can help you.

A close friend of mine has been looking wonderful these days. She's in her mid-forties, her skin glows and she's been receiving even more compliments than usual on her looks these days. She credits this to her healthy eating habits, regular spa sessions and time spent at the gym. Yes, that has played a part, but I think there's more to it, because my friend has always been disciplined. I believe the reason for her luminous look is an unacknowledged one. Love. After exiting a marriage that hadn't been making her happy for a long time, she's now in a relationship with a man who adores her. She finally has the love of a good man, who celebrates her and treats her the way she deserves to be treated.

Love looks good on all of us. At our core, we really want very few things—to be loved, to be wanted, and to belong. We seek these feelings throughout our lives and find solace in our various relationships and within ourselves.

There is strong evidence that good relationships contribute to a healthy and happy life. Study after study has shown that good interpersonal bonds only benefit our lives. People with strong social relationships are 50 per cent less likely to die prematurely.[1] Researchers have also found that people who completed a stressful task experienced a faster recovery when they were reminded of people with whom they had strong relationships. Those who were reminded of their stressful relationships, meanwhile, experienced even more stress and higher blood pressure. In fact, a survey of 5,000 people conducted by the National Bureau of Economic Research in the US found that doubling one's group of friends had the same effect on one's well-being as a 50 per cent increase in income.[2]

But why do good relationships impact us in such a drastic way? Well, no one is an island. Some are the high and mighty tides at night, some are the shells on the sandy beach, some are the birds flying far away from sight, some are the rocks that brace the harshest of weather, but all of this have come together to create the island. We depend for our well-being on a balance in our relationships. This quality is the foundation of our society, and it is in the very core of our DNA to interact, unite and overcome challenges together, and survive and strive together. The positive energy of good relationships flows to correct the balance within us and helps us feel complete. It is through this balance that we connect with others. But, on the other hand, if a relationship is negative in some way,

[1] Julianne Holt-Lunstad, Timothy B. Smith and J. Bradley Layton, 'Social Relationships and Mortality Risk: A Meta-Analytic Review', *PLOS Medicine*, 2010, https://journals.plos.org/plosmedicine/article?id=10.1371/journal.pmed.1000316 (accessed on 28 July 2020).

[2] John F. Helliwell and Haifang Huang, 'Comparing the Happiness Effects of Real and On-line Friends', The National Bureau of Economic Research, 2013, https://www.nber.org/papers/w18690 (accessed on 28 July 2020).

it will disrupt the balance within and not only affect that one relationship but other vital foods too.

Do you remember the movie *Cast Away*? Tom Hanks's character is stranded on an island and is so desperate for human company that he makes a football his friend. His compulsive need for company was what stayed with me long after I left the movie theatre.

Our important relationships not only include family and friends, but also meaningful connections with our bosses, colleagues, employees, house helps and pets. A healthy relationship can be shared between any two people who love, support, encourage and/or help each other. People in healthy relationships listen to each other, communicate openly and without judgement, trust and respect each other and make time for each other. In such relationships, each person grows and encourages the other to as well. They focus on 'us' and 'ours', and not 'me' and 'mine'.

We know why relationships are so important to us. Why, then, are we unable to overcome the unhappiness we feel about certain people or because of their presence or absence in our lives? The most common roadblock to good relationships, in my experience, is the ego. The ego is, essentially, who we believe ourselves to be. It is an identity that is constructed by us and not true or objective at all. We base it on what we think we deserve rather than on what we might actually deserve.

An egotistical person's self-worth is driven by external factors, mostly validation from others. People with big egos are often insecure and try to cover up their shortcomings by pretending to be important or better than everyone else. Such people tend to lack confidence and self-love. One of the first signs that your ego is in the way of a healthy relationship is the tendency to blame the other person. Carefully examine if there's an unwillingness to see a situation from the other's perspective. Every time there is a fight, do you find fault or blame someone else? Or vice versa? If you find yourself thinking that it's never your fault or you're always right, consider that this might be your ego speaking.

I was invited to a party recently, where the host told me that she'd only invited people who talk to each other. Those who didn't get along with any one of the guests didn't make the cut. I found her thoughts a bit immature, as people should always be willing to put their egos aside, especially when they are older and more mature. When you are on a path of total well-being, one of the first things you need to do is kill your ego. Why wreck relationships when you can nurture them and be a happier, more content person?

That is exactly what I constantly strive to do. I was anyway not one to hold on to grudges. And with time, I have become more aware of the need for fulfilling relationships. This has automatically laid my ego to rest for good. Even when I know I have been in the right after a silly argument with someone, I make sure the other person doesn't take it personally. And if they have felt slighted, I apologize immediately. Contrary to what a lot of people believe, this trait is a gift, not a weakness. It's wise to at least try to be the bigger person and work on the relationship rather than walk away, vowing to never speak to them again. People with egos are just not happy. They can even break relationships with the people who have loved them for years. But at what cost? Just so they can believe they have won the argument?

Indulging your ego can only lead to negativity in your life and create a vicious circle of ill feelings. We as human beings need to stop looking at situations from angles of strength and weakness. Putting your well-polished and diamond-crusted ego aside may make you feel weak at first, but remember that many external things will always make you feel lesser anyway, and certain people will let you down at some point. But you need to realize that true happiness lies in forgiving and forgetting, regardless of the wrongs that have been done to you. Stay true to yourself, and what you stand for. Let people call it weakness, but I promise you that you will always be known as that one person with the most genuine smile and the kindest heart in every room you step into.

The Secret to Strong Relationships

I have been married a long time. I also have friends who have been part of my life for many years now. I am proud of the people around me and the effort all of us have put into making sure our relationships have been strong and enriching.

The key, I have learnt, is communication. Relationships don't exist in a vacuum. When two people come together, they bring their own past experiences and expectations with them. Over time, these expectations can strain a relationship, and you may feel like the other person doesn't care because they are not acting the way you think they should. The only way to understand the other person in the relationship is by talking to them, understanding what they want and then making sure your expectations align.

People tend to confuse talking with communication. They believe that if you talk to your partner or meet your friends often for lunch, you are automatically communicating.

But it goes much deeper than just talking and hearing what the other person has to say. It is also about paying attention, getting your point across clearly and truly understanding the other person's perspective. By asking questions like 'How are the kids?', 'How is your work?' and 'How is your mother?', you may not really be communicating. Most people listen so they can respond with their own stories, not to understand.

Without being a good listener, your relationships won't prosper. To listen, you have to develop a genuine interest in the other person. Be curious about their point of view, rather than just trying to have an answer for everything. I'd also recommend Atticus Finch's timeless advice: 'You never know a man until you stand in his shoes and walk about in them.' All of us are fighting battles every day that others—sometimes even those closest to us—don't know anything about. Empathy goes a long way in saving relationships. That is why if you've had a tiff with someone close, instead of lashing out or sulking, ask yourself a few imperative questions, and if you can, the other person too: What is causing them to behave the way they are? Why did they say what they did? Is there something you don't know about that's really bothering them? Have you done something wrong for them to react in a hurtful manner? Answering these questions will give you an insight into the minds of those you love.

Your relationships flourish when you are able to be yourself and can speak your mind without being judged by the other person. Hence, it is wise to refrain from telling the other what to do. My husband and I are very different people. I am an organized person and want a clean house and everything in the right place. But my husband's work desk is messy, with coffee cups and paper strewn around. Sometimes, I tidy up the desk, but a few hours later it is back to being the way it was. While I am always on time for all my work and personal appointments, he never is. Luckily for him, he cracks a joke and everyone forgets that he was late. He is a night person, while I sleep early. I love salads, but he hates even the lettuce on his deep-fried burger. All of these traits used to bother me early on in our marriage. But not any more. My journey on the path to absolute balance has taught me to accept my husband as he is. My criticism clearly wasn't working—it rarely does—and we would only end up arguing the rest of the time. All those traits are part of his personality, just like the other traits I love—he is a good person and a wonderful friend, son and father. It's not right for me to only love him for his good qualities, is it? I slowly began to accept the parts of him that I didn't always agree with. Now we have a genuine relationship, where both of us are happy, even though I do my best to hide the burgers when I can. When you accept another person's flaws, you grow to love them even more. None of us is perfect. In fact, the things you find perfect about yourself, the other person could think of as imperfect. By accepting my husband's flaws, we have reached a place where he accepts my flaws too.

No marriage is perfect. Ask your grandparents and parents—they'll tell you how they have lived through the sensitive phases of their togetherness. The heady romance fades away after a few years, and marriage becomes more about companionship and friendship, and fighting over who has to get out of bed and switch off the lights before sleeping. People get misled by fairy tales, and think that's how their marriage will always be. They expect more than the partner can give. They compare their relationship with those of their friends and feel they are lacking, not realizing that everybody and every relationship is different.

Marriage is about sticking it out. It's about not quitting based on your mood. I grew up believing that the vow of marriage was sacred. When I said, 'To have and to hold, from this day forward, for better, for worse, for richer, for poorer, in sickness and in health, to love and to cherish, till death do us part', I meant these words with all my heart. And I have lived by them. These vows tell us that we have to support each other through good times and bad. Of course, no one should tolerate violence, and mental and physical abuse. But fighting with your partner and leaving the marriage for seemingly petty reasons is not fair to either party. Several studies have shown that being married to a good partner can have a lifelong positive effect on one's well-being, including helping one weather the dip in life satisfaction that comes with middle age.[3] Happiness is even higher among couples who see their spouse as their best friend. This happiness, from a healthy, fulfilling relationship, permeates to other parts of your life too and can bring peace and joy to those relationships as well. When the people in your life make you smile, and you make them smile in return, it creates a bond of friendship that asks for nothing in return but love, and promises to always shower you with eternal joy and laughter. This completes the circle of life.

---

[3] John F. Helliwell and Shawn Grover, 'How's Life at Home? New Evidence on Marriage and the Set Point for Happiness', The National Bureau of Economic Research, 2014, https://www.nber.org/papers/w20794 (accessed on 28 July 2020).

The No-Negativity Challenge

Friends are sometimes as important as spouses in our lives. According to Dr William S. Pollack, assistant clinical professor in the department of psychiatry at Harvard Medical School, 'Our brains and bodies function best when we are part of a community and maintain close, personal connections.'[4] Friends help us deal with stress, make better lifestyle choices that keep us strong, and allow us to rebound from health issues and diseases more quickly. Relationships usually are mirrors that show us the ways in which we need to change and become better friends. Our friends and the people we have long-term relationships with allow us to be vulnerable and ask for help the way we normally wouldn't with strangers.

But, as we all know, friends don't always come in packages we like. I have had all kinds of friends—energy vampires, selfish, generous and loving. Over the years, I have developed a radar that tells me how to spot a long-lasting friend from a fair-weather one. It has served me well, and I have rarely been proven wrong. But that still doesn't mean I will treat them differently. I get along well with everyone because I accept everyone for who they are. I don't criticize them. Pointing fingers only drives people away. I always give people many chances; I don't believe in cutting people out of my life just because they have let me down with their behaviour a few times. That's their journey and they have to live with themselves. They will learn and change themselves

---

[4]   'A little help from your friends', *Harvard Health Publishing*, Harvard Medical School, 2016, https://www.health.harvard.edu/staying-healthy/a-little-help-from-your-friends (accessed on 30 July 2020).

if given enough time. It is natural for us to criticize and judge others, but it takes a strong person to step back and keep their distance. *Be that person.* Lots of people give others just one chance, and if they fail, they don't forgive. How can you build lasting relationships this way?

Love the people in your life just as they are. Humans are hardwired to notice the negatives first. Break that pattern. One of the best ways to do that is to try what I call a thirty-day zero-negativity experiment. If that sounds overwhelming, begin with the pledge that you'll do it for a couple of days.

Be mindful about not seeing negativity in anything you encounter. Try not to judge. When you notice a negative thought, consciously bring your mind to a positive thought. Look at everyone with love, understanding and empathy. Appreciate them for who they are. Once you start this, your perception of things, people and life will start changing. Your conversations and actions, interactions and connections will evolve. Live and let live is the mantra you have to live by. Tell yourself that just because you have given birth to children doesn't mean you own them. Just because you have married someone doesn't mean you can control them. Just because you're someone's friend, they don't have to give you all their attention. Once you put this into practice, I know your life will change for the better. So try to adopt this mindset for two days. If you feel good at the end of it, extend it to thirty days. In no time, it'll be your constant state of mind.

How to Fight Right

My live-and-let-live attitude has meant that aggressive confrontation has never been part of my life. It was only later, when I was learning about spirituality and calmness of the mind, that I realized how my personality is suited to resolving conflicts. I have always believed in having a quiet, non-accusing conversation to confront issues bothering me or the other person. Confrontation in relationships should never be done with the purpose of bringing down the other person. Making them feel small and triggering their anger by talking down to them never ends well.

The best way to fight is to choose the correct words to convey what you're feeling. Be careful what you say when you are angry, because words once spoken can never be taken back and can haunt the rest of your relationship.

Never say . . .

- 'You never . . . ' or 'You always . . . '
- 'I'll talk to you when you can be rational.'
- 'We're done! I'm out of here.'
- 'You're such a @#$%&.'
- 'Why are you making such a big deal of nothing?'

Instead, say . . .

- 'Please try to understand my point of view.'
- 'I can see my part in this.'
- 'What are we really fighting about?'
- 'Let's take a break for a few minutes.'
- 'We should stop and think about this, rather than letting it escalate.'

By choosing positive language, you will allow the discussion to end fruitfully and not with both of you stomping away from each other. Sometimes, we focus so much on what we want to say that we forget to think about how we're conveying it. And, more importantly, what our body language and expressions are communicating. Learn to manage your expressions and your body language so you don't come off as aggressive. Instead, strive to be someone who wants a positive outcome from the argument. Make sure there is no tightness around your mouth and eyes, and you don't frown, scowl or glare at the person. Pointing and jabbing at the other person, keeping your arms and legs crossed and fists clenched, and encroaching on the other person's space should also be avoided. Instead, relax the muscles around your eyes and mouth, nod and have open hand gestures, and uncross your arms to look understanding and accepting. Learn to understand that at moments such as these, it isn't your rational mind speaking, it's your ego. We regret most of the things we say in anger because we don't genuinely mean them. So at such times, learn to calm yourself down and let that egotistical moment pass. With time, you'll realize that 99 per cent of the things that triggered that egotistical side were not half as bad as you initially thought.

I know that the temptation to yell at someone is strong when things aren't going well during the argument, or in the relationship in general. But if we only knew what happens to our bodies when we are in such a situation, we would avoid yelling at all costs. When we have reached a place where we're shouting at someone else, the body is stressed. Once the stress response engages, the prefrontal cortex of the brain, which is responsible for decision-making and planning, starts to shut down. The emotion centres of the brain's limbic system take over, and instead of thinking carefully, we are driven by what we feel. That makes it incredibly difficult to really process what the other person is saying in an objective way. In essence, we stop being able to hear each other or come up with appropriate responses, and the hurt that comes with the yelling stays with both of us as a deeper, significant memory. What's worse is that it takes at least twenty minutes for the chemical released during the stress response—cortisol—to leave the body. That is a good chunk of time before you can talk calmly again in person or over the phone, and you're at risk of saying and doing things you might regret later on.

Compare that to what happens when both you and your loved one are discussing the issue at hand in a calm, peaceful manner. Your breathing is calm and your muscles are less tense—you will most likely not hurt the other person by what you say and how you say it.

I have dealt with problems in both ways, and I can say for sure that the second one is much easier on you and the person you're disagreeing with. I reached that stage, thanks to my journey towards balance and accepting that the only thing in my control is my reaction to a situation. Why choose something that ends up harming my body and my relationships? When we don't have happy relationships, we don't function as we are meant to. We break, we fall apart, we ache and we hurt others. The absence of love and belonging will always lead to suffering.

Fear and anxiety are hard to avoid altogether. Healthy relationships foster well-being because they make this fear and anxiety more manageable. Unresolved distress activates the fight-or-flight response. The long-term flood of stress hormones affects the immune system and even our ability to think and learn. It's the healthy relationships that help us regulate our emotions, calm our primal alarm systems and promote longer periods of health. They are a safe place to manage our worries, fears, hopes and dreams.

Before I end this chapter, I want you to go back to the circle of life and examine what score you gave to relationships. Now list down the specific relationships you want to improve, and what exactly you can do for each to make them better. The approach towards a friendship may be very different from what you need to do to make things better with a parent. When you think about your close relationships calmly and rationally, you will understand them better and even learn to deal with them in a more productive manner.

HOME ENVIRONMENT

Home and heaven are one.

What do you most look forward to when you have had a long, gruelling day, when the world doesn't feel like a good place, the safe haven you thought it was? When it feels like you're at odds with everything and everyone around you? I know what I yearn for on such days. Home.

Just like love, home is a four-letter word that carries with it emotions that are hard to put into words. A song from a forgotten American movie, *Country Strong*, comes closest to describing how I feel about coming home. The song talks about home as a place where you heal when you are hurt, where you will always be welcome, sheltered in the toughest times till you can recover and rejuvenate from the stress of the outside world.

Home is a place that's filled with the people you love; it's where you are always supposed to feel safe, accepted and loved. I have been lucky enough to have been born in, and later married into, such a home. My family and home are like warm blankets on a cold night that I can rely on. I know that no matter how harsh it gets out there in the world, we will be all right.

Not everyone is fortunate to have only good memories associated with home. But it's still possible to create something that feels like your special place. Moreover, it's the people that contribute so significantly to making a home. Sometimes, you may find more love with people other than the ones you thought you were supposed to find love with. Home is usually associated with a place, but in reality it is a feeling of warmth, comfort and safety, which also stems from the relationships you have with the people you live with. Sometimes you have to search for a place you can call home, and sometimes it finds you. It could be a mansion or a small room, but if you feel love and warmth, you are home.

The impact of a loving home environment on emotional well-being cannot be overstated. The quality of love a person experiences at home affects them from infancy through adolescence and into adulthood. Children need stable, supportive social environments, where their needs are met, to enhance their cognitive, emotional and physical development. Unstable, noisy and chaotic home environments have negative effects on children's health. These can significantly shape habits and attitudes in adulthood and can hold people back from realizing their full potential and living their best life.

Research shows that a negative home environment during a child's first three years results in a host of developmental problems, including poor language development, behavioural problems later in life, and aggression, anxiety and depression.[1] That is why it is so important to build a home that helps

---

[1] G.W. Evans et al, 'Crowding and Cognitive Development: The Mediating Role of Maternal Responsiveness among 36-Month-Old Children', *Environment and Behavior*, 2010, https://journals.sagepub.com/home/eab (accessed on 28 July 2020).

children thrive, because an unhappy child will grow up to be an unhappy adult.

Are You Living in a Toxic Home?

A lot of times people don't even know they are living in an unhealthy home because that's all they have known. For them that is the norm. Living with people who are a negative influence on your mental health is a burden you should never have to carry. Watch out for these signs to know if you grew up in or are still living in a toxic home.

- *You feel invisible:* A family that neglects your needs damages your mental health and self-esteem. It's easy to feel invisible when your parents and siblings act as if they are too busy for you. You may feel like nobody seems to care how you are doing and what you are feeling. Instead of communicating openly and honestly, your family makes you feel isolated and insignificant. If your partner's or parents' needs are always put before yours, it is a sign that you are living in a toxic home. When you try to voice your concerns, they may tell you that you are being preposterous.
- *You feel pressured:* Does your family impose conditions on you? Do you feel loved and accepted by someone only when you live up to their expectations? Indian parents are particularly guilty of this. They have a tendency to believe they are doing it for your good, but their behaviour can quickly become toxic when they criticize every little mistake you make and have unrealistic

expectations of you. Even when you know things aren't going well, your parents or partner will remind you how lucky you are to be living with them.

- *You feel trapped:* If you feel like you come home only because you have no choice, you need to examine your relationship with your family. You would like to leave, but you are made to feel guilty or ashamed for wanting to do so. Sometimes you even lie just so you can get away from them, even for a short time, and you feel relieved when you do so. If you feel compelled to lie about your family to your friends, spouse or colleagues, it is not normal.

- *You feel unhappy:* If you are more unhappy around your family than happy, your home environment is unhealthy. A lot of times, toxicity builds over time and you reach a point where you can no longer bear to be at home because of all the negativity it adds to your life.

Make Your Home Emotionally Healthy

An emotionally stable home provides security, a place to grow and the foundation for a happy, healthy life. No family gets it right all the time, because we are humans. We goof up and unintentionally hurt the people we love. But that doesn't mean we shouldn't try to reach for the ideal—a home where every family member knows that their feelings matter and that they will be cherished and loved, no matter what. All healthy families have certain things that all members should try to imbibe:

Sharing feelings: Make time to listen to others and validate each other's feelings. If someone is facing a crisis, put aside your own feelings for just ten minutes to hear them out and help in any way you can. Allow all sorts of emotions to be expressed, even if they are hard to hear. All family members should also show affection physically. When you hug someone, you tell the other person you love them and you care. I am a big believer in the power of the human touch. It is a component of health and stress reduction that is usually underappreciated. Science has shown that touch, massage, hugs and any physical acknowledgement in general help release feel-good hormones that keep us relaxed and stronger in the face of stress.[2]

Parents working as a team: In every family, one parent is always more lenient than the other. In my house too, when my kids were growing up, I was the one to lay down the rules, while my husband was the more indulgent parent. Such a situation can get unhealthy if either parent refuses to budge from their stance. So my husband and I decided that despite our different parenting styles, we would always present a united front. That way, neither of us would feel resentment for the other, and the kids would know what the boundaries were.

Not tolerating abuse: People in emotionally stable homes take responsibility for their thoughts and feelings, and

---

[2]   Maria Henricson et al, 'The Outcome of Tactile Touch on Oxytocin in Intensive Care Patients: a Randomised Controlled Trial', University College of Borås, 2008, https://onlinelibrary.wiley.com/doi/abs/10.1111/j.1365-2702.2008.02324.x (accessed on 28 July 2020).

are aware of how their actions affect others in the family. The household has clear rules that everyone is expected to follow, such as never using abusive language with one another. In such a home, emotional and physical abuse is never tolerated. A home where one or two people have all the power is an abusive and toxic home. Even if it doesn't happen every day, it adds great stress and casts a shadow on the home. The connection between an abusive home and stress cannot be emphasized enough. People, especially children, who have been emotionally, physically or sexually abused, experience trauma. It leads to the build-up of fear, uncertainty, anger and frustration over time. A person who is under constant stress sees danger everywhere and security nowhere. Such a person tends to react without thinking in most situations, committing acts they may regret later. The body responds to stress as though it is in danger. That is all right once in a while, but always being in stress mode drains one physically.

A study conducted by the University of California, Los Angeles (UCLA) found that toxic childhood stress alters the neural response to stress.[3] This boosts the body's emotional and physical reaction to any sort of threat and makes it more difficult for that reaction to be shut off. People who are emotionally, physically or sexually abused can become hardwired to overreact to circumstances and stresses later in life.

---

[3] Judith E. Carroll et al, 'Childhood Abuse, Parental Warmth, and Adult Multisystem Biological Risk in the Coronary Artery Risk Development in Young Adults Study', *Proceedings of the National Academy of Sciences of the United States of America*, 2013, https://www.pnas.org/content/early/2013/09/18/1315458110.abstract (accessed on 28 July 2020).

Giving each other space: When you share a physical space with someone, it's important to adjust to each other's habits and preferences. This can be done by having honest, heart-to-heart conversations with them to avoid conflict and maintain harmony. At the same time, make it a point to give each other emotional space too. Don't always hover around the other members of your household. Everyone needs privacy, freedom and alone time to grow and flourish. It allows you to reflect, grow and nurture yourself. I spend at least a couple of hours by myself every day. Whether it's for work or relaxation, I enjoy my own company. Each of us in the Panday household has our favourite corner and knows not to disturb each other at certain times.

Purge a Few Things from Home

Constant conflict has no place in a happy home. Some habits and attitudes are triggers of conflict that *need* to be eliminated—or, at least, severely reduced—so that every family member's well-being is taken care of and prioritized.

- *Screaming:* Screaming always begins as a one-off event and ends up becoming the norm. It happens without anyone even noticing that people at home are constantly screaming at each other. In some homes, that is how people tend to communicate most of the time. Screaming also often leads to violence. A study at Harvard Medical School revealed that screaming can permanently alter the brain structure of an infant exposed to it regularly.[4] It affects the

---

[4] 'Excessive Stress Disrupts the Architecture of the Developing Brain', Center on the Developing Child, Harvard University, 2014,

integration between the two parts of the brain, which can cause personality problems and affect emotional balance as the child grows older. The best way to fight this is to implement a no-scream rule at home, which everyone has to follow, without exception.

- *Hostility:* Do you feel like your family members don't want the best for you? That they are resentful towards you and express it every chance they get? Living among hostility isn't good for your mental health and self-confidence. There are homes where family members are not enthusiastic and where people rarely smile. If you identify with this and find it difficult to relax at home, it is probably not the best situation for you. You deserve a chance to live with people who cherish you.

- *Drama:* We all know people who create drama in all kinds of situations. But when they are your friends, it is easier to handle because you don't live with them. It becomes difficult to live with family members who look for problems, not solutions, and only focus on the negative aspects of life. This pessimism is contagious and makes you feel distressed and frustrated. In such a scenario, try to maintain a positive attitude and let such people know that their attitude is harming others at home.

I have encountered my share of drama queens and kings in my life, which has encouraged me to be calm and composed. It is tough to handle such people, though. But after decades

https://46y5eh11fhgw3ve3ytpwxt9r-wpengine.netdna-ssl.com/wp-content/uploads/2005/05/Stress_Disrupts_Architecture_Developing_Brain-1.pdf (accessed on 28 July 2020).

of practice and years of yoga and meditation, I know how to react to such tantrums. The best way to deal with any sort of drama in your life is to stay silent at that moment, sleep on the issue and discuss it the next day or whenever you find the appropriate time for it. You can also take a few deep breaths to calm yourself so the situation doesn't escalate. If that doesn't work, just remove yourself from the situation and go for a walk. You'll feel much better afterwards. I find that I rarely get angry—probably once a year—because I'm mindful of my feelings.

- *Chaos:* Our surroundings affect out mood. When we are out in nature, we feel calmer and at peace. Similarly, if we spend most of our time in an unorganized and chaotic space, it can lead to mental chaos and stress. In such environments, our brains have more difficulty processing information, and that affects our productivity and increases anxiety and stress. This is not about just the physical space but also chaotic communication and disharmony among family members. An uncluttered and clean home invites positive energy and doesn't eat into your mental and emotional energy.

The Physical Space You Call Home

A neat and organized house is the first step to having a wonderful home. The average person spends about 87 per cent of their time indoors, so it makes sense to create a space around you that you love. A clean home keeps bugs away and reduces allergies caused by dust, thus contributing to your health, which can have a significant impact on your mental well-being. I start to clean my home when I get angry or stressed about something. Concentrating on cleaning diverts my attention, and in some time, I feel calmer and less stressed.

Living in an uncluttered home also helps reduce distractions and improve concentration. In fact, organizing your home, especially your pantry, can make you more aware of your food and spending patterns. You may realize that you buy a lot more food than you need or stock up on too many packaged snacks. Being aware of what is in your kitchen will also help you cook at home. We'll go into this more in another chapter.

Being in a home where the dishes are left in the sink, children's clothes are strewn across the bedroom floor and where the living room has become a playroom often has a negative impact on you that you may not even notice. It is much harder to find things when they are hidden under a pile of clothes, or even concentrate on tasks at hand when there's a lot of stuff in your way. Emotionally, it makes you ungrounded, as this set-up doesn't offer a suitable space for you to relax and unwind after a long day. The mess takes over every room, leaving you without a space to call your own. Physically, you may get tired, as the stress of living in a cluttered home often manifests as aches and pains throughout the body.

Let's consider an example. You probably have a job where you work long hours. When you wake up in the morning, tired from the previous day, you've snoozed your alarm three times and are in a hurry. You try to look for the black shirt you wanted to wear to your meeting today, but it takes you an extra ten minutes because it's buried under a pile of clothes you never got around to putting away in your cupboard. You rush through breakfast, leaving the plate and your coffee mug in the sink, thinking you'll come back and do it. You get caught in traffic and are late for the meeting. This upsets the rest of your day's schedule and you leave work late again.

You're tired when you get back. You step through the door, and see the mess you left in the kitchen, which sours your mood. You go to your bedroom and realize you never picked up your wet towel from the bed and left the dirty laundry on the floor in your rush to leave. It just makes things worse. You want to exercise, but as you dig into the mess, you know it'll be a task to find your workout clothes, so you plop down on the bed, where the sheets are damp from the towel. You close your eyes, exhausted. Later, you do the bare minimum—and it all repeats the next day. Sounds familiar? The only way to break out of this cycle is to carefully look around your home, acknowledge the problem and slowly chart out a plan to tidy up. Don't attempt to do all of it in one day—it'll just be overwhelming, and you'll want to give up midway. Set yourself small goals and tasks, and keep ticking them off your list till you're satisfied that your home is the neat and tidy place you want it to be. As you keep doing that, also think of how you can customize it to your likes and dislikes. Here are some suggestions on how to imbue positivity into your surroundings.

Fill your home with houseplants: Indoor plants are a great way to purify the air, boost your mood, improve your health and sharpen focus. They are considered an important part of feng shui, as they contribute to the positive flow of energy throughout the house. Just close your eyes and think about it. When you're outdoors, in a park or a forest, surrounded by greenery, doesn't everything feel fresh and calm? Is that an atmosphere you would like to replicate in your home?

There are plenty of houseplants that don't require too much attention. If you have the space in a balcony or a front or backyard, consider growing some on your own, right from planting the seeds. It can become an educational experience that can relieve stress and also be fun. You'll learn new gardening techniques and have the health benefits of fresh herbs, say, basil and coriander, which are easy to grow and might even save you some money. If you have a bumper crop, you can even share it with your family, friends and neighbours. Also, by opening up your windows and letting fresh air in, you will bring a lot of positivity into your home. We use a lot of artificial lights through our gadgets, so we need some natural light as well every so often.

Take out some time to be one with nature, and you'll realize how much more relaxed you feel. It's where we belong, not in small little cubicles that cut the cord that connects us to nature. Whenever you have the chance, sit by a window, on a verandah or in your garden, and take in the chirping of birds, the song of the crickets and the swaying of the trees.

Get a pet: The Panday home has a dog, a cat and some fish, and we love them all so much. Animals are known to help with depression, anxiety and stress while also providing companionship and easing our loneliness. Now that my kids are more independent and don't need me as much as they used to, I spend a large part of my free time playing with my adorable puppy, Peach. I have so much fun playing with him, and he truly lights up my life. Our cat, Cappuccino, is also playful but in the understated way a cat is, very unlike the unstoppable energy of Peach. Every creature is different and has its own beauty. Cappuccino doesn't express love in the same way Peach does, but he has an air of calm that I really like. It's important to remember that every single person or animal has a different kind of beauty. You just need to look at them without expecting something in return, and you'll be able to find it.

Play music you love: I love listening to all kinds of music, especially when I am working out. Music has the power to uplift and change our mood. Try to listen to different kinds of music and see how each influences your mood. You'll find yourself gravitating towards certain songs, bands or genres, and that's perfectly fine. That's the kind of music you really connect with. When we were redecorating our home, I wanted speakers in many corners of our house so we could have lovely music playing in the background throughout. My husband, however, wasn't in favour of the idea, so we shelved the plan. But if given a choice, I'd still opt for that.

Keep mould at bay: Indian homes also tend to have a lot of leakage issues. Moisture is a common problem in bathrooms and sometimes even in the living areas. If the moisture level is too high, it could result in mould growing. People who are sensitive to it can have reactions such as sneezing, runny nose, red eyes and skin rashes. Keep checking for mould so your family isn't in harm's way.

Keep chemicals away: I sincerely hope no one smokes in your family, because having cigarette fumes in the house sucks out the positivity from a home. Other than its disastrous effects on the family's health, tobacco smoke also mixes with the air in your home, making the quality of the air you breathe poorer. The particulates in the smoke also settle on walls, furniture and flooring. I'd also recommend using organic aromatic oils instead of the ones that are laden with chemicals to have a lovely, clean home environment. And it's best to stay away from fragrant air fresheners that come in a spray can because they mostly comprise of chemicals. The easiest way to get some clean fragrance in the house is scented candles. Find an aroma you like, leave them on in every room to feel fresh and relaxed.

Also, keep the use of pesticides inside the house to a minimum. Overusing pesticides at home can lead to nerve damage, skin irritation, headaches and nausea. I am a firm believer in eliminating as many chemicals as possible from your home. There are plenty of natural remedies that you can use to clean your home. I have listed a few below:

a. *White vinegar:* Vinegar is a natural disinfectant. Since it's acidic, it's great for getting rid of rust and hard water stains.

b. *Baking soda:* It absorbs odours in the air. Use it in litter boxes, garbage cans and diaper pails to keep the stink down. Sprinkle it on a damp cloth to use as a gentle surface cleaner on counters, sinks, ovens and stoves.

c. *DIY cleaner:* For mild cleaning, mix 1/2 cup vinegar, 1/4 cup baking soda, and 4–8 cups hot water in a spray bottle. For a stronger solution, use 2 tablespoons borax, 1/4 cup vinegar and 2 cups hot water. Add a few drops of essential oil to any mixture to give it a fresh scent.

d. *DIY glass and mirror cleaner:* Combine 3 tablespoons vinegar with 4 cups water for a mild cleaner. Make it stronger by using vinegar and water in a 1:1 ratio; or 1/4 cup vinegar, 2 tablespoons cornstarch and 4 cups warm water. Wipe with a microfibre cloth, then do a final wipe with a dry cloth to avoid streaks.

e. *DIY kitchen sanitizer:* Combine 1 cup vinegar, 1 cup club soda and 2 drops tea tree oil. Spray it on to surfaces and wipe clean. This mixture works to disinfect only if it's made fresh.

f. *DIY microwave cleaner:* To get rid of food odours or hardened food splatters in the microwave, mix 6 tablespoons baking soda or 1/2 cup lemon juice with 1 cup water in a microwave-safe glass container. Microwave the mixture until it boils, then leave it inside with the door closed until it cools. The steam will loosen the grime and make it easy for you to wipe the inside of the microwave.

g. *DIY drain-pipe cleaner:* Put 1/4 cup baking soda down the drain followed by 1/2 cup vinegar. Cover and let sit for fifteen minutes; then uncover and pour in 8 cups of boiling water.

h. *DIY toilet cleaner:* Mix 1/4 cup baking soda with 1 cup vinegar and pour it into the toilet bowl. Let it sit for three to thirty minutes, scrub with a toilet brush and flush.

Get an air purifier: The first step to good health is to make sure you're breathing in clean air. Air pollution significantly affects each aspect of our health. Fine particulate matter has been linked to lung and heart issues, which, in turn, can lead to other complications. Invest in a good air purifier to mitigate the risk. You can also use sage smoke, because it is known to clear up airborne bacteria and disinfect the air. It also releases negative ions, which is known to put people in a good mood.[5]

Purify your water: A water purifier cleans tap water and makes it fit for human consumption by removing chlorine, chemicals, pesticides, heavy metals and bacterial contaminants.

Declutter your living space: If you take a little time every day to pick up after yourself, you'll get in a bit of exercise and allow yourself the mental space to focus on how you actually want to spend your day productively. Plus, if your home is in order, you'll be more open to inviting friends and family over spontaneously. The more clutter you have in your home, the more cluttered your mind will be. Ask yourself the questions below when you are decluttering your home:

    a.   Have I used this item in the past twelve months?
    b.   Am I keeping this because I am worried about wasting money?

---

[5] N.T.J. Tildesley et al, 'Positive Modulation of Mood and Cognitive Performance Following Administration of Acute Doses of Salvia Lavandulaefolia Essential Oil to Healthy Young Volunteers', *Physiology & Behavior*, 2005, https://pubmed.ncbi.nlm.nih.gov/?term=%22Physiol+Behav%22%5Bjour%5D (accessed on 17 August 2020).

c. Am I keeping this because it has sentimental value?

d. Does this sentimental item hold me back?

e. If I were seeing this item for the first time, would I buy it now?

f. Do I have other items that serve the same purpose?

g. Do I plan to use it in the near future?

h. Is this broken thing really going to be fixed?

i. What can I do with these items?

Hang pictures everywhere: If you are looking to seek inspiration and motivation from your home, consider hanging art that you resonate with. It should inspire, stimulate the mind and be pleasant to look at. Artwork has been shown to encourage creative thinking, boost self-esteem and increase brain connectivity.[6] Include pictures of family and friends throughout your home. The pictures we choose to frame are often of us living a happy, carefree life, where we feel loved and supported. Such photos can boost our mood and serve as reminders to create more picture-perfect moments. You can also put a cute welcome mat at the door, which makes your guests and visitors smile and feel welcome into your cosy home.

Place flowers everywhere: Nothing says cosy like flowers. Flowers make the home look more colourful, welcoming and homely. Spread them out around your house and notice

---

[6] Deanne and Gary Gute, 'How Creativity Works in the Brain', National Endowment for the Arts, 2015, https://www.arts.gov/sites/default/files/how-creativity-works-in-the-brain-report.pdf (accessed on 28 July 2020).

your face break out in a smile every time you see them. If you find them too expensive, you can get some fake ones as well that look inviting.

Paint walls: Another way to brighten up your home is to paint the walls. Look into different colours and styles that you may like. If painting the walls is a cumbersome exercise that may affect you financially, hang tapestries or wallpaper for some creativity and fun.

Create a cosy sleeping space: In the chapter on health, we will discuss the immense importance of getting enough and quality sleep. Here let's focus on where you sleep. You can begin your healthy sleep routine by creating a space that is as comfortable for you as possible. Invest in sheets and blankets that you love and that are well suited to the weather. If you have a window in your bedroom, hang shades or curtains that block light from outside seeping in while you're asleep. In the morning, take time to make your bed. Not only is it nice to come home to a well-made bed, but it can also give you a sense of accomplishment first thing in the morning. These simple steps can improve the quality of your sleep, which directly affects your overall health and vitality.

Store food in glass containers: Use glass containers to store your food. Plastic contains toxic chemicals that can wreak havoc on your hormones. Plastic leaches toxins into food, which can have terrible effects on us and also destroy our environment. Glass is infinitely reusable and recyclable.

Add a silent room: If you have a spare room in your house, designate it as the 'silent room'. Ideally, it should be located away from street noise. If you don't have the space, put up a folding screen so it can serve as your spot. Of course, there should be no TV, no audio and no mobile phones. This can be a place for everyone in the family to sit without distractions and concentrate on themselves. A prayer room can also double as a silent room. I have a similar room at home too. It has black walls that relax us and calm our senses. We use the room to read, meditate, work on art, nap or just work in general. It's also a technology-free space, where all of us can go to for some me time. If you have space, add a rocking chair in a corner of the silent room, or any other room. That can be your personal space to chill, put your feet up, read a book and relax. Your silent room can also double as a mini library. Books make a home look and feel cosy, and they will be the perfect accompaniment to your rocking chair.

Do over your bathroom: Your bathroom can also serve as a space where you can have some me time. A few fluffy towels and candles will create a spa-like atmosphere, especially if you can find some space to add a bathtub.

Explore feng shui: Feng shui is an ancient Chinese philosophy that focuses on the connection we have with our environment and how it affects our overall well-being. It is believed that the flow of one's energy in a space is what makes an environment healthy. Certain principles of feng shui, such as using calming colours, positioning your bed correctly and using curved furniture, are believed to promote rest and relaxation. Some feng shui tips include:

a. Fixing any leaks at home, as they represent financial leaks.

b. Incorporating photographs or paintings of flowing water, running horses or moving boats at home, as these represent money flow and abundance.

c. Keeping the stove clean, as it represents abundance. Also all burners should be used equally. Utilizing each burner opens up a variety of opportunities and financial channels.

d. Choosing wooden bed frames, as metal frames attract electromagnetic waves from technology and affect sleep cycles.

e. Paying attention to the airflow in your living space. Put in fans for air and energy movement and plants for air purification.

I hope this chapter helps you focus on what is most important in this world—your home and your family. Creating a stress-free, beautiful space that you and your family can come home to after a long, hard day is in your hands. In the fast-paced world we live in, creating a happy and healthy home is an achievement and accomplishment, and will go a long way in creating balance in your life. I can assure you that the moment you improve this aspect of your life, a lot of other things will become easier and start falling into place too.

Tech at Home

During the pandemic, our homes turned into literal sanctuaries and kept us safe from possible infection and, worse, death. This time has only increased the importance of a good home environment for us. While people were complaining about having to make the most of a limited space and about getting on each other's nerves, what came to our rescue is technology.

We live in a hyperconnected world, and that term has got a bad name of late. It has led to no downtime and people have been accused of living their lives online more than in the real world. The stress of this hyperconnection has been affecting a lot of people, which is why so many people now talk about social media detox and have no-tech hours and rooms in their homes.

But technology was our saviour during the lockdown. It kept a lot of people sane during those turbulent times and gave them an outlet for their feelings. Our entire world shifted online. People worked, attended classes, met friends and family, and conducted financial transactions online.

Technology has many pros and cons. It gives us so many ways to save time, access information, manage our finances better and communicate more effectively. But it has also made us more dependent on our devices. These also come with security and privacy concerns. Ironically, they have led to a sort of social disconnect. Our mental health has suffered too as a result of the constant stimulation we are subjected to.

The lockdown showed us that there was an urgent need to balance out the use of technology in our lives. While it was a blessing during the quarantine period and self-isolation, technology has also been a curse to many of us. It is only by balancing the time we spend on it that we can make optimum use of it. By doing so, we reap its benefits and stay away from the havoc it can create. Here are a few ways you can manage technology:

- One of the best ways to digitally detox is to step outside and make the most of nature and the outdoors. There are so many beautiful things around us that we fail to notice because we are busy on our phones. So keep gadgets aside when you're out of your home and drink in the best that nature has to offer.

- We need to digitally detox inside the home too at times. Begin by turning off notifications and alerts that are not important. That way you won't check your phone as often as you usually do.

- You can also put your phone on airplane mode when you're working out or playing with your kids. These activities require your full attention, and there shouldn't be any distractions at such times.

- In my home, we have a rule that everyone will keep their phones away during meals. A similar rule can be instituted when you're out having dinner with friends. Phones should be kept in bags or pockets, so everyone is truly present at the table.

- Set an alarm for social media usage. I've set an alarm for an hour on Instagram, so I don't exceed the time I spend on the app, even though I mostly use it for work. I also make it a point to not binge-watch any TV shows. I know it's tempting to continue with the next episode even past bedtime, but it's unhealthy for my sleeping pattern, so I turn it off after a couple of episodes and continue the next day.
- Finally, always ask why when you pull out your phone. If the answer is boredom, you need to find something better to do with your time. Read a magazine or a book, or talk to your family members when you feel like checking your phone too often.

FINANCES

Hello willpower, hello billpower.

Like all parents, mine, too, have enriched my life with the lessons they have taught my siblings and me. The Woodham family was a fun, loving and simple unit, which always had its values in place. My three sisters, two brothers, parents and I lived in a 2 BHK flat in the posh Pali Hill neighbourhood of Bandra in Mumbai. We were surrounded by neighbours—many of them from Bollywood—who had access to the best material things money could buy, while we stayed in a company flat—thanks to my father's job as a packaging director for an advertising agency—with no telephone or car, and a black-and-white television that arrived much later than our neighbours'. But we made up for it with heaps of love and laughter, and our strong values.

Growing up, I didn't realize that my family wasn't as well off financially as those in our locality. Now when I look back, I realize they used to travel abroad regularly for vacations while we didn't even have bicycles. At a time when our birthdays were celebrated with new stitched dresses from the local tailor, samosas and jalebis for snacks, and Kismi toffees as return gifts, the kids in my neighbourhood had clothes bought during trips abroad, lavish birthday parties with entertainers and fancy return gifts. But none of this mattered then. I realize only now that there was such a difference between us and our neighbours. In fact, we were one of the last families to have a television. I remember the day we got the black-and-white TV. We were all so excited and spent days watching Doordarshan. Every Sunday, we'd go to church, have a family lunch, finish our homework and then sit in front of the TV to watch the weekly movie that would be telecast.

Simple is the only appropriate word I can use to describe our family and lifestyle then. My father was friends with some of the residents of a nearby fishing village and often took us to their weddings and birthday parties, where we danced with abandon. The year I was in Class 2 stands out as a particularly memorable one. As usual, we received one egg each on Easter and crackers to burst on Diwali. Our father also dressed up as Santa Claus to give us small gifts during Christmas. That year, my father was gifted a few tins containing twenty to thirty packets of biscuits for which he had designed the packaging. We were so ecstatic to eat as many biscuits as we wanted that my mother was sure we would fall ill. We happily shared our biscuits with our neighbours, who were used to eating imported chocolates.

We also learnt about the importance of saving. In the 1970s, in Bandra, vendors would go door to door selling vinegar in huge glass bottles that were 4 feet tall. One day, my father got home an empty vinegar bottle and turned it into our piggy bank. Into it, we would put all the spare change left from our pocket money after buying sweets such as jeera goli and candy floss, because my father had told us that one day when we had saved up a lot, we could use it to buy whatever we wanted. A couple of years later, we bought lots of toys at the Bandra fair using the money from that piggy bank, which would otherwise have been tough for my parents to afford. It was such a lovely, happy day.

My father worked hard to provide us with the little luxuries of life. We could have easily thought of that time as one where we didn't live like our Bollywood neighbours, but those are not the values we grew up with. Without telling us in as many words, my parents taught us that what truly mattered in life was the joy we found in what we had without hankering for what we didn't. We learnt by example that money could never be a substitute for love and hard work and that true happiness is almost always found in the simplest of things. Most importantly, I learnt that less was always more—and that's a lesson I have never forgotten.

My own journey as an adult seeking financial independence began a couple of years after marriage. I remember that a few years ago, I was featured in an article in a women's magazine about how I made my first million. To say I worked hard to have a bank balance of my first Rs 10 lakh would be an understatement. Months and months of dedication, perseverance, passion for my work and some good business and financial decisions led me to that glorious moment. But it didn't follow easily and was peppered with its own set of challenges. Only once you see failure do you truly understand the role money plays in this world. Being one of the first few independent female gym trainers at the time, my journey was not only difficult but also financially impractical. Few feelings match up to the knowledge that you are an independent person in every possible way. Financial independence gave me more confidence and the courage and determination to follow my dreams, and have an unassailable say in my own life.

My biggest takeaway from my decades-long career has been that if you put all of yourself in the work you do, the rewards can be remarkable. The second thing it has taught me is the importance of financial freedom and having one's finances in order.

Managing your money is a lesson that will benefit you your whole life. It requires, first, a willingness to take responsibility. You have to have a basic understanding of personal credit and pay your bills on time so you don't suffer from debt. Financial independence is also about accepting that sometimes you have to sacrifice immediate wants for long-term gain. All of that requires budgeting, saving, protecting those savings and spending wisely. If this sounds daunting, it's understandable. I feel the same way. In such a scenario, hire a trustworthy expert to do what you can't. Not everyone has to master the ability to handle their finances themselves. Even if you understand it theoretically, it can be tough to apply it in real life. Back in my younger days, I had a rule: NEVER buy anything you don't need on a daily basis. It sounds strict, but when you're working to make ends meet, you have to make every rupee count.

To be truly financially free means having the ability to not let money, or the lack of it, get in the way of happiness. For that, you should know how much you make and how much you spend. The first step is to make a list of your assets and everything you owe. When you subtract your liabilities (what you owe) from your assets, you will arrive at your net worth. This amount has to grow over time. If your net worth is stagnant or shrinking, you should re-evaluate your investments. These investments should appreciate as time passes. These thumb rules are non-negotiable and are the only way to ensure your financial health is secure.

Another rule that all experts recommend is a consistent savings and expenses pattern. Twenty per cent of your income should go towards savings, 30 per cent towards activities and purchases you want, such as restaurants, concerts, travel and shopping, and the remaining 50 per cent should be spent for basic facilities, such as food, housing, transportation and bills.

Financial Freedom and Happiness

These are practical tips everyone should learn and implement. And yes, while it is important to have enough money to survive and thrive, I firmly believe that happiness and contentment have nothing to do with bank balance. The idea that someone richer than you is also happier is a fallacy. Similarly, believing that once you are worth a certain amount, you will automatically be happy is also wrong.

Happiness is a state of mind, and it is within your control, irrespective of your financial situation. What matters more is financial freedom. When you achieve that, you start living a self-determined life. Most people live a predetermined life, where they spend most of their time working to earn the money they need to build a better lifestyle. The little free time they get is spent on family, errands and other personal needs. This leaves very little free time to create a unique life destiny. Basically, you work throughout the week for forty years and try to have fun with what little time remains.

All that changes when you achieve financial freedom, which could mean that you have enough money to follow your passion and still be able to take care of your loved ones and other responsibilities you may have. It can put you in the unique situation of being able to take away all the stress that comes with being bound to a job or situation that pays the bills. And even when you reach that stage, you shouldn't forget where you started from, and the work you had to put in. Most people start to take it easy at this stage. When I first made money, I never looked at it as something that could be spent. Instead, I thought of it as a marker of how far I'd come. While being true to myself and my goals, I always made sure I reminded myself that there was a long way to go.

Achieving financial freedom is beautiful, but it also requires a lot of work. Just remember to always look at your financial patterns and learn from them. Evaluate the good decisions, but also what went wrong. When it comes to money, we need to listen to our mind, not our gut. We need to make sure we make the right calculations.

For a stress-free financial life, you need four things to fall into place:

- Control over day-to-day and month-to-month finances.
- The capacity to absorb a financial shock.
- Being on track to meet financial goals.
- The financial freedom to make choices that allow you to enjoy life the way you want.

The most important takeaway from this is that when we handle money wisely and give it an appropriate amount of significance in our lives—not too little, not too much—it makes us happy. While I was researching for this chapter, I came across the '100 Thing Challenge'. People around the world took part in it. The idea was to reduce possessions in one's lives to the bare minimum—just 100 in this case—that could contribute positively to one's life experiences, and to get rid of everything else. It worked on the belief that the ability to purchase things is not what happiness is based on—it is our life experiences that bring us that feeling. It makes me incredibly happy to know that people have begun to actively lead lives that lead to happiness, instead of believing that it comes with objects or things. Our relationship with money need not revolve constantly around buying new things and feeling less stress and more security when we are able to do so.

Remember that financial freedom is more important than wealth. If you spend more than what you earn, it doesn't matter whether you are rich or poor—you aren't financially free. There is a wonderful quote from the movie *Fight Club*: 'The stuff you own ends up owning you.' Life is so much more than just accumulating things. How will you ever be content if your yardstick of happiness changes with evolving fashion trends?

Everyone has a different idea of being financially free. It may be the freedom to choose a career you love without worrying about money, or the freedom to take an international vacation every year without straining your budget, or the freedom to help those in need. Decide what it means to you and work towards it accordingly.

Become Financially Secure

Here are a few ways I recommend you start your journey to becoming financially free and self-reliant.

1. *Record your expenses:* The first step to start saving money is to figure out how much you spend in a

month. Keep track of all your expenses, even if it's a coffee at Starbucks. Organize the numbers by category—such as petrol, groceries and loans—and total each amount. Use your credit card and bank statements to make sure you're accurate.

2. *Budget for savings:* Once you have an idea of what you spend in a month, you can start budgeting so you can plan your spending and limit overspending.

3. *Find ways to cut your spending:* If your expenses are so high that you can't save as much as you'd like, it is time to cut back. Cancel subscriptions and memberships you don't use, especially if they renew automatically. Reduce the number of times you eat out and cook more often at home. It will also contribute to your health and you will save substantially. You can also give yourself a cooling-off period. When you are tempted to buy something you don't really need, such as one more handbag, wait a few days. You may be glad you passed. Or first save up for it.

4. *Set savings goals:* Set short-term and long-term goals. Then figure out how much money you will need and how long it will take you to save it. Short-term goals include an emergency fund, which has three to six months of living expenses, vacation or down payment for a car. Long-term goals can be down payment on a home loan, your child's education and your retirement. Also, invest in a good medical- and life-insurance policy, so if you ever need to visit a hospital, you don't have to worry about the bills.

5. *Pick the right tools:* You can choose from fixed deposits, stocks, mutual funds, government bonds and much more. Consult an expert before you start investing.

6. *Pay off credit cards in full each month:* The miles and cashback offers are only valuable if you're not falling into debt or paying interest. Timely bill payments will also ensure that your credit score remains high.

7. *Save automatically:* By setting up an automatic savings account, you won't have to worry about the hassle of saving at regular intervals. This will come in handy on a rainy day.

8. *Start saving for your retirement:* Few people get rich on a salary alone. You build wealth due to compound interest over many years. Start on the fun as soon as you start earning, because young professionals are in the best position to save for retirement.

9. *Put your bills on auto-pay:* This ensures they are paid on time, so you don't end up paying late charges.

10. *Have a spending limit for gifts:* We don't realize how much we end up spending on gifts for our family and friends. They don't always need a thing from you to know that you love them. Actions always speak louder when it comes to showing love. Maybe you can decide to give gifts only on birthdays and festive and celebratory occasions. This will surely relieve you of financial stress. Flowers, a home-baked cake, or a card with loving, heartfelt words will always carry more meaning than a shopping voucher.

11. *Have a no-spend day:* How about choosing one day a week you decide to not spend any money on anything that is not necessary? That one day can be allotted for free family-and-friends fun. Cook at home and plan free activities such as a game night, watching a movie or going to the park.

12. *Say no:* A big part of saving is also learning to say no to yourself and to others for expenses that aren't essential. Many people pay for things because of ego and esteem. It's perfectly fine to split the bill sometimes.

13. *Dream of a financially free future:* Picture yourself in the future, with all of the things you've ever dreamt of beside you, and understand that you can't get there by spending all of your income. You get there by saving it and using it wisely. I know that off-white shirt looked great on you, but, trust me, there'll be plenty of time for that.

If you are still unsure about certain aspects of your financial situation, answer the following questions. They will give you a better idea of the steps to take.

- If money were no object, what would you change in your life?
- What are your top financial worries?
- What are the three smartest financial moves you've made?
- What do you consider your three biggest financial mistakes?
- When in your life were you happiest? What made it a happy time? And what role did money play in it?

- What's the minimum amount of money you need every month to keep your financial life afloat?
- If you were out of work, how long could you cover expenses before having to take drastic financial steps?
- What did you learn about money from your parents—and which of these beliefs have you adopted as your own?
- Think of three people you know who are in great financial shape. What have been the keys to their financial success?
- Is it important to you to drive a nice car? If so, why?
- In the typical week, which moments do you enjoy and dislike the most?
- Is getting rich one of your overriding life goals?
- Think about your weaknesses. Are they acceptable human failings or are they inflicting major damage, including major financial damage?
- Who depends on you financially? And how would they cope if you suffered an untimely demise?
- When is it okay to go into debt?

The Karmic Flow of Money

I am an independent professional. I conduct workshops on balance. My income depends on how many people sign up for my workshops. In the course of my work, I have encountered many people who try to negotiate the fees I charge for my work. I understand the need to secure a good bargain, but what people don't realize is that by doing so, they are disrespecting my experience and what I have to offer. That is why I ensure I know my worth and charge fair rates. By doing so, I keep the karmic flow of money going. In fact, when other independent professionals like me don't charge sufficient rates, they break the karmic cycle.

We expend our energy when we work. Charging rates that are in alignment with the service you provide helps you live a life of financial strength. This allows you to create balance in your life, work with interesting clients and still have the time for fun.

One of the biggest things that will impact your financial freedom is your career. Choosing a career you love, excelling at it and making sure you are earning what you and your talent deserves are things you should keep in mind. There is no reason to stay stuck at a job that is making you miserable. By finding a job that you enjoy, you will support your goals of financial security. In the process, every day will be a fun adventure that you can't wait to get started on. Your work should allow you to grow creatively and financially. Choosing a career that has income-earning potential becomes important here. So even if you're not making your dream salary from the beginning, ensure that there is scope for your income to increase as your value increases.

Financial freedom is about more than just being able to cover unexpected emergencies without feeling the stress. The fun begins when you realize you can fulfil your needs as well as that of your family. Remember that you don't have to be rich or have to wait until you reach some level of achievement to enjoy your life.

Eat Well on a Budget

A nutritious diet certainly can be expensive, but it doesn't have to be. Use the following tips to cut costs on your grocery bill.

- *Make a plan:* Know what you plan to cook during the week and how much you'll need. That way you will only shop for what you need with a few buffer items in case plans change. You will also not purchase more than required. Otherwise, unused food can end up spoiling and getting thrown away. That is not only waste of money, but also waste of food.

- *Make a list:* Know what you're going to purchase before you get to the store. Grocery stores are designed to entice us to purchase more. So you can end up adding a significant cost to your grocery bill.

- *Shop for local, seasonal produce:* Food that is in season is available in large quantities and hence cost less. You will also do your bit for the environment, because seasonal food is locally grown and will not travel a long distance to reach your plate.

- *Buy in bulk:* If you have the space to store it, buying bulk food is always cheaper than buying single items.

CAREER

Tough times don't last; tough people do.

Every day at 6 a.m., my alarm rings, which I've set to a soothing song I love. I open my eyes, paying attention to the familiar tune. Rested and happy, my face breaks into a smile. I stretch and get out of bed, looking forward to the day.

After breakfast, I head to my happy place—the gym. I then look forward to starting an exciting work day . . . My career is my ikigai. Ikigai, a Japanese word, is composed of two words: 'iki', which means life, and 'gai', which describes value or worth. According to the Japanese, everyone has an ikigai. An ikigai is essentially 'a reason to get up in the morning'. It has four characteristics that come together in one thing—what you love, what you are good at, what the world needs and what you can be paid for. Thankfully, the work I do as a wellness coach is the perfect combination of all of these things for me.

I sincerely hope the current job or career you are in is your ikigai too. If not, is there any activity that you always turn to when you have to relax? Something you can imagine not getting tired of, which you can lose yourself in and completely enjoy?

We spend most of our waking hours at work. That is why it is imperative to spend those hours doing something you love. You know about my journey to reach where I am today. I studied to become a commercial artist, but found my passion in fitness. It was a profession where I knew no one. But I started small, by writing articles, and was soon offered the chance to train Miss India contestants. Since then, there has never been a day that I have woken up unhappy about going to work.

Do What You Love, Love What You Do

A few years ago, I worked part-time as a personal trainer. It gave me immense joy to guide someone to achieve the body they wanted. One morning, ten minutes before I was meeting a client at the gym, I had a little accident where I cut my hand on a piece of glass. It was hurting a bit, and I probably needed stitches from the looks of it, but I didn't want to miss out on an hour of fun. So I cleaned the wound, put a band aid on it and went to the gym. My client was shocked when she saw that my finger was bleeding. I told her I wasn't feeling much pain, that I just wanted to get on with the workout, but she didn't listen to me and insisted that I go to a doctor. I finally gave in. The stitches on my finger still remind me of that day. The scar helps me feel gratitude at having found something I love so much. I was willing to work through the pain because I knew the joy would eclipse it. The Greek have a word for this: *meraki*. It means to put something of yourself into your work. It is all about the soul, creativity and love.

Doing what we love completes a vital part of our lives. It gives our journey meaning and brings us a sense of responsibility and belonging.

When you love the work you do, you never work a day in your life. Work becomes fun, and it is no longer the tedious thing you have to do to fill up your day and earn a living. Working in a job you don't love can take a toll on your mental health. If your Sunday nights are always filled with dread in anticipation of another week of work, it's worth taking a deeper look at your work and career. In such a scenario, you *have* to figure out what it is that adds meaning to your life and if there is a way to make it work for you. I'm not saying you need to just give up everything you've worked towards, drop it all overnight and take up something you love. That choice is up to you, and you should think clearly about how it would affect you and others around you. There are a lot of factors to consider.

But I can assure you that doing something you love will bring a wave of joy and peace into your life. You'll have a strong sense of purpose, enthusiasm and no dread waking up and going to work every day. If what you do is taking a toll on you physically and mentally, to a point where your world is crumbling around and within you, maybe it is time to chart a path to a career you will enjoy. At first it will be tough, but if you've truly found where you belong, that commitment and drive will push you way further than you have gone in any other job. We're always scared of change because we look at the effort it took us to get here, but change is the only way we can grow, and change is what got us here in the first place.

To know which job is right for you depends on your preferences and goals, and not what everyone tells you is the perfect job. Remember these points to understand your true passion:

- The right career choice will lead you to greater happiness and success.

- The best jobs are those that you love to do and which also give you ample personal time. Such workplaces will not suffocate you, and employees tend to stay on in such jobs even if it doesn't pay them the money they'd like. This is because they are happy with the way things are going for them.
- The right job will make you feel happy in whatever you do, and you will also be satisfied with your contribution at the workplace. This will happen specifically through a career that helps you enhance your skills and learn new ones as you grow in your job. So the right career is not only about a salary. Playing an important role in the office is much more satisfying than a handsome paycheque from a workplace where you don't contribute much.

Many people spend decades in careers that are diametrically opposite to what they actually want to do in life. The correct balance in life happens when you find work you love or learn to love the work you do. Also, you don't necessarily have to leave your 9-to-5 job to have a fulfilling career—there are other ways to find gratification. Here's how you can work through two of the possible scenarios you face.

a. How to Find the Work You Love

- Make a list of your strengths and interests. Think of how you could turn them into an inspiring career. Get creative.
- Think about the things you end up telling your friends and family about—it could be how you love to trek every weekend, how proud you are of

the little garden you've built in your balcony, how you look forward to redecorating your home every couple of years, or even the intricacies of the legal system, to those who are interested.

- Research the career options you have narrowed down for yourself. Gather information on the paths you are considering, and how they could influence and shape your goals.

- Reach out to professionals working in that field. They can give you information, support and guidance about possible opportunities and pitfalls.

- Join professional organizations or attend social events to create authentic connections, and make yourself visible as an expert in the field.

- Contact prospective employers to learn about potential career opportunities. Be professional and enthusiastic, and remember that even if a company isn't hiring, it's never a bad idea to send them your résumé.

- Be patient. Finding a new career that you love may take time. You might have to try a few jobs before finding an ideal fit.

- Close your eyes and think about the things that have brought you the most happiness and joy until now. Maybe it was you going up on stage in Class V to dance on your school annual day or playing a part in the college play. If those few minutes on stage made you feel like the king of the world, maybe that is where you belong, and always have. Not because the world believes that, but because you do.

b. How to Love the Work You Already Do

I understand that not everyone may have the opportunity to change their career when they want to. It could be because of family, financial or logistical reasons. In such a scenario, it is easy to feel demotivated and you can even come to hate your job. Before you reach that stage, I have a few recommendations. Try them out, and I'm sure you'll feel better about going to work.

- Request to work on projects that interest you. Tell your employer or supervisor about the areas or kind of work you're passionate about. You are likely to put in more effort if you enjoy what you do. That's where you will see the best results.
- Surround yourself with peers and colleagues who support your work.
- Accept constructive feedback and work towards improving your weak areas.
- Stay motivated by giving yourself small rewards for accomplishing goals, such as short massages, long walks—think vital food.
- Make your office environment more attractive. Add fresh flowers to your desk and hang motivational quotes and pictures on the soft board or around your desk. Make your workspace an expression of yourself. This is where you spend a large part of your day. If your desk makes you feel sluggish and bland, fill it up with things that evoke creativity and motivation.
- If you are going to move to another position or company, make sure you've considered the quality of

work too. Seek fresh opportunities that satisfy your
desires, and always maintain business relationships
with previous employers.

I believe the first indicator that you are in a job that doesn't
excite you is when you don't look forward to going to work
at all. Sure, everyone has Monday blues, including me. But
when you're having Tuesday and Wednesday blues as well,
maybe it's time to find a job or career that works for you.
You know you are in the wrong job when you move from
one to another in quick succession. It happens because
you are searching for the right job but end up somewhere
wrong again—and the chain continues. The simple fact
may be that you are not happy with what you are doing.
If you are switching fairly often only for a better salary,
you're not considering the work you do. You're spending
time and energy in searching for new jobs when you could
be using them to find your true passion. In the long run,
it could harm you, especially if you're in a small industry
with not many companies to switch to. Instead, if you
invested that commitment into one job, it would probably
make you far more successful, and money would follow.
To be successful, you don't have to find better-paying jobs—
you have to find the job that you're willing to put your
life into.

Find Your Ikigai

We have all been put on Earth for a purpose. That purpose
is not to sit in an office you don't like. Actor Harrison Ford
was unsatisfied with the kinds of roles and opportunities
being offered to him. So he took a new direction in his

career and became a self-taught carpenter. He continued this profession for fifteen years as a way to support his wife and children. But one day he got a call to audition for director George Lucas. He then went on to play the role of Han Solo in *Star Wars*. And, of course, he's never looked back since.

So if you've been following your dream, but it hasn't led to your dream job or the perfect opportunity, don't give up yet. You only fail when you've given up completely. If you are skilled at something and keep putting yourself out there, it will get noticed and could lead to incredible opportunities. What needs to stay intact is your hope, your belief and your interest. The good things in life don't always come easy, but, with time, things do fall in place—you just need to keep going and learning. People who don't stop always reach their destination.

Brandon Stanton started an Instagram page we all love, called Humans of New York. He used to be a bonds trader before he took up photography. He had no prior training, but his passion led him to start interviewing passers-by on the streets of New York. He discovered that this was the most fulfilling and energizing way to spend his days. He found his ikigai.

To find the ikigai in *your* life, I have come up with a few questions you can ask yourself:

1. What do you love doing? Write down the first thing that pops into your mind.

    *   What can you not stop talking about when you're not working?
    *   What would you do even if you weren't getting paid for it?

- What activity makes it feel like time is flying and you aren't getting bored?

2. What are you good at?

   - What do your friends and family come to you for advice on?
   - What are you proud of?
   - Does developing your skills in this area excite you?

3. What can you get paid for?

   - Is this something people would pay for?
   - Can this give you the income you desire?
   - What does the competition look like?

4. What does the world need?

   - What kind of contribution to the world would you like to make?
   - Will there be demand for it in ten to twenty years?
   - What larger impact could you have by doing this?

I love that in the process of finding your ikigai, you also have to take a deeper look at your whole life and work towards setting different aspects of it right.

To make the right career move, do an honest evaluation of your skills. You may think you're a good cook, but you could actually be a mediocre one. Ask a professional in the field or your family and friends to give you an honest opinion of your skills. Maybe all your friends tell you that you make delicious Italian food and that you should consider a career in it. But Indian food could be closer to your heart. In such matters, knowing you're a good cook helps. But what will help you more in your career is if you know what exactly you like about cooking. Finally, every job should not only make use of your talent but also enhance it. As a chef, you should know everything there is to know about cooking—the terminologies, the intricacies of the cuisine, etc. The real secret of life is to be engrossed in what you're doing. Instead of calling it work, you will realize it is actually play.

Fight the Fear

Making a transition is scary, disruptive and difficult. Research on stress shows that the brain biologically perceives changing jobs as a life change that poses a threat to survival. In fact, the Holmes–Rahe stress scale found that making a career change is one of the twenty most stressful things that can happen in your life, just behind the death of a close friend.[1]

Dreaming of becoming a successful chef when your degree and skills are in marketing cannot be easy. Financial responsibility is a factor that you are likely to consider. The key, then, is to start small. If you're currently in a job you dislike, use your spare time to experiment with your

---

[1] 'The Holmes–Rahe Stress Inventory', https://www.stress.org/wp-content/uploads/2019/04/stress-inventory-1.pdf (accessed on 29 July 2020).

interests and passions. Once you are confident of your new path, think of giving up your regular job. Actor Ken Jeong, whom we know from the *Hangover* movies, was a practising physician. He discovered acting in college and did short stand-up sets every few months, even when he was busy. He continued his day job as a doctor, but kept performing and auditioning, landing roles here and there. He only gave up medicine full-time after he struck it big with the first *Hangover* movie.

You may have to invest in retraining or spend some time earning less than you'd like, as you're entering the workforce as a beginner. But as long as you're not spending beyond your means, you should be financially secure. In time, and with the right skills and work ethics, you should be able to earn enough to live comfortably.

There is fear, however, beyond financial commitment. It's scary to redefine your identity in the professional world: What if I fail? What if I am bad at it? What if I send out 100 résumés and not get a single interview? These questions can paralyse you and stop you from taking that first step. But the only way to be true to yourself, live the life you've always dreamt of living and finding that career balance is to face the fear head-on. How do you know you will fail if you don't even take that first step? We tend to build up failure in our minds and think of the worst possible scenario as the only outcome. But this is your career, something you will be doing for at least forty years of your life. The least you can do is give a different career option a try. That way you won't live with regrets. My mantra is to always try something and hope it works out. Take baby steps before the big plunge and see how well those pay off.

Did You Know?

Anna Wintour was fired from the fashion magazine *Harper's Bazaar*. She could have let that impact her career and life. But she didn't give up and has been the editor-in-chief of *Vogue* since 1988. She is considered to be the most powerful woman in fashion. She says getting sacked was one of her most important learning experiences.

Passion Trumps Money

For a lot of people, money means happiness. I do not discount the importance of money in anyone's life. We need it to survive and live the life we have always desired. It gives us a sense of security and peace of mind. But only money in the bank can't do that. The right career also contributes to peace of mind. Just running after money without being happy at work is no good. Similarly, working in a job you love where there is no scope of earning enough is also not a wise idea. That is why we need to strike a balance between money and work, as well as the other things mentioned in this book.

Following your passion will see money following soon. It may not be there on Day 1, but you will eventually earn the salary you deserve. Here are a few reasons I would rate passion over salary.

- You can relate more to the work you do and come up with better ideas. Being forced to do a particular job is one of life's most draining experiences. While there are times where you may find the work tiring and dull, you'll get past them. Your creative process will also be different. You will be more inclined to come up with creative ideas when you like what you do.

- No matter how much money you make, nothing will help you overcome the feeling of doing something you hate. Many people enter corporate life and put in crazy hours during the week for a great paycheque. They may have plenty of money saved up, but never really get to enjoy the fruits of their labour. In such a scenario, you only end up hating your job because you don't really care about what you do. This lack of energy and negativity will also be a barrier to finding happiness.

- When you really enjoy what you do, nothing will stop you from getting your work done and achieving success. You feel unstoppable because your passion and interest give you the energy to work.

- Our careers will consume most of our lives, so we might as well do something we enjoy. Once you realize this, you will lead a happier and more fulfilling life.

How to Become an Entrepreneur

Do you stay at home but yearn to have a career? If you are unable to become a working professional, why not start your own business, even if small? You get to be your own boss and make decisions about what you do, how much money you make and what hours you put in. Ideally, you can work on your business on weekends when the responsibility of housework is not yours alone.

I know someone who chooses to stay home to take care of her son. But she is an excellent baker. She would bake cakes on all of her friends' birthdays, who kept urging her to start selling her baked goodies. After years of dilly-dallying, she finally took the plunge. She started baking on weekends and when her son was at school. She looks happier now—there is a spring in her step. The confidence has worked wonders for the other aspects of her life as well.

However, starting a business can be overwhelming. The key to overcoming this is to have clear vision and being organized. Focus on what you can do now and how you want your business to look today. Close your eyes and imagine yourself owning your business. What days and hours do you work? Cultivate a business mindset. To be successful, you need to believe you are a successful business owner. Your interaction with potential clients, business partners and marketing contacts will benefit from your ability to speak confidently. Be professional, concise and courteous in your conversations, and reach out to people to start networking.

You don't have to be an extrovert to start connecting with people. Simply be yourself.

Here are some ways to start:

- Remember that every person you meet can become a potential client.
- Collect contacts and be in touch.
- Step out of your comfort zone.
- Share your excitement about what you are doing.
- Be genuinely interested in others.

Acknowledge the protective internal voice in your head, but decide that you're not going to let it control your actions. When you're in a job you dislike, it's easy to stay put and accept the steady paycheques. Making the move is then a risky proposition. But that will only lead to more frustration and dissatisfaction in your current job.

You are meant to shine, so that others see you and follow your path. I highly recommend doing what you love for a living, because it is the best antidepressant you will ever get. A career of your choice won't leave you fatigued or stressed. There is ample research to show that stressful jobs lead to poor eating, which, in turn, causes a lot of physical issues, which can have an impact on your mental health. It is a vicious circle that you have to break out of. Happiness in your career is an important part of the circle of life, because everything in life is connected. A good career fit impacts your life satisfaction. If the shoe fits, you'll love wearing it.

How to Achieve Work-Life Balance

- *Learn to say no:* Don't feel bad about saying no. If it's too much for you and your well-being, just say no politely. Self-care always comes first.

- *Stop checking your email:* Learn to be present in the moment. Checking emails after work can increase your stress and anxiety levels. Also, in most cases, you can't really do anything until the next morning when you reach work anyway. So why fret?

- *Leave work at work:* Set boundaries for yourself. Before leaving work, write a to-do list for the next day, so you can forget about work while enjoying your me time. Also make an effort to be more actively engaged at work. That way you'll get more done, and peacefully be more present at home too.

- *Fit in something in your day that you enjoy doing:* This can dramatically improve your well-being and mental health. By having something to look forward to, you can improve your happiness and productivity, and decrease stress levels.

- *Get enough sleep:* Not getting enough sleep can impact you. The right amount—between seven and eight hours—will increase your energy levels both at work and at home. You are also less likely to be cranky.

- *Don't fret over what you can't control:* Make a deliberate effort to stop yourself from stressing over things that you have no control over at the moment, such as a submission or the rude tone your boss adopted while telling you something you didn't like. Negative thoughts that linger on even after you have left your workplace will only lead to additional stress, whereas positive thoughts will keep you looking forward to your days of work ahead. Spend your free time wisely and in the company of good people and good thoughts.

HEALTH

Self-care is the new healthcare.

Imagine waking up to the best view in the world. You open your eyes, sit up and smile at what's in front of you. For someone it could be their partner. For someone else, it could be their pet at the foot of the bed. I love waking up to the view of beautiful natural landscape—green and lush—in all its glory.

That is what I woke up to every day at The Farm at San Benito in the Philippines, a wonderful detox centre I visited at the beginning of 2020. I visit a couple of detox centres a year because I live in a polluted city like Mumbai and need to get away from all that it does to overwhelm my system. The air in the city is full of pollutants, such as smog, cigarette smoke, metal ions and radiation. These generate free radicals that exist in the atmosphere alongside pollutants in the air. These free radicals affect our body in many ways. They have been linked to central nervous system diseases, such as Alzheimer's, cardiovascular disease due to clogged arteries, inflammatory disorders such as rheumatoid arthritis and cancer, ageing of skin, hair loss and diabetes.

And it isn't just pollution that wreaks havoc on our bodies. The pesticides we ingest from the food we eat, the toxic effects of the many plastic products of our everyday life and the chemicals that we apply on our skin and hair from beauty products make the situation worse.

That is why I recommend a regular detox programme that helps flush out these toxins from the body. Some people invest in expensive handbags, and others in luxurious vacations. I invest in my health. It could be anywhere the air and water are clean, and where I have a chance to eat organic or farm-grown healthy food.

There was a wide array of tempting and inviting treatments to choose from at The Farm. They included programmes for weight loss, anti-ageing, beauty, aesthetics, dental treatment and body rejuvenation, among others. However, I chose the detox programme, which concentrated on one of the most neglected organs of the body—the gut.

Everyone has their own definition of good health. For some, it's about looking great, for others it's about weight management through exercising and dieting. And all of these goals are valid, because different people have different priorities. For me, good health is about beauty inside out. And that begins and ends with a healthy gut. Yes, exercising and eating the right foods are always a priority for me. But these have little meaning if my gut is not in order. From everything I have learnt about good health from my experience and the books I've read, I have realized that if one's gut is not in good shape, the rest of one's body won't be as well. In this chapter, I'm going to focus on this vital aspect of physical health. My other books, *I'm Not Stressed* and *Shut Up and Train!*, delve into other facets of how to keep the body and mind healthy. You'll soon see how the gut has a direct or indirect impact on so many body functions, and understand why I picked it as the main topic for this chapter on health.

Trillions of bacteria and microorganisms live in our bodies. Most of them thrive in the small and large intestines and are responsible for essential tasks to keep us healthy. Since your gut bacteria line your intestines, they come in contact with the food you eat. This may affect which nutrients you absorb and how energy is stored in your body. Studies have shown that gut bacteria are one of the things that decide the degree of weight loss after you follow a certain lifestyle.[1] In another study, when gut bacteria from obese people were injected into mice, the mice gained weight.[2]

One of the most important bacteria in the human gut is *B. theta*. It is a bacterial species found in people who enjoy fibre-rich diets and maintain a healthy weight. In overweight and obese people, *B. theta* are often scarcer.[3] The gut bacteria can influence how fats are absorbed in the intestines, which also affects how fat is stored in the body. They alter how we balance levels of glucose in the blood and respond to hormones that make us feel hungry or full.

Most books talk about general health without paying much attention to the gut—the most important component

[1] Serguëi O Fetissov, 'Role of the Gut Microbiota in Host Appetite Control: Bacterial Growth to Animal Feeding Behaviour', National Library of Medicine, 2012, https://pubmed.ncbi.nlm.nih.gov/27616451/ (accessed on 30 July 2020).

[2] Vanessa K. Ridaura et al, 'Gut Microbiota from Twins Discordant for Obesity Modulate Metabolism in Mice', National Library of Medicine, 2013, https://pubmed.ncbi.nlm.nih.gov/24009397/ (accessed on 30 July 2020).

[3] Erica D. Sonnenburg and Justin L. Sonnenburg, 'Starving Our Microbial Self: The Deleterious Consequences of a Diet Deficient in Microbiota-Accessible Carbohydrates', National Library of Medicine, 2014, https://www.ncbi.nlm.nih.gov/pmc/articles/PMC4896489/ (accessed on 30 July 2020).

of good health. This chapter will tell you everything you didn't know about your gut and how, with a few changes in your lifestyle, you, too, can make it healthier and happier.

What Exactly Is the Gut?

The gut is the second brain of the body. That is because it has as many neurons connected to it as the spinal cord. The gastrointestinal tract transports food from the mouth to the stomach, converts it into nutrients and energy, and passes waste out of the body. The gastrointestinal system, however, has a more complex role in our bodies. Apart from digestion, it has been linked to various health factors, such as immunity, emotional stress and chronic illness, including cancer and type 2 diabetes.

A healthy gut can help you improve your overall health, energy levels and fight off diseases, mostly by properly absorbing healthy nutrients and eliminating bad ones. The most common reasons that people now suffer from gut problems, particularly inflammation, is eating too much unhealthy food, the presence of harmful food additives, excessive consumption of antibiotics, excess sugar in the diet, the presence of unhealthy bacteria and the lack of beneficial ones. This inflammation results in a weakened immune system, which increases your chances of falling sick.

It All Begins with the Microbiome

The key to a healthy gut is the microbiome. The gut microbiome is made up of trillions of microorganisms and their genetic material that live in our intestinal tract. Inside us is a mini world that has a life of its own.

These microorganisms, mainly bacteria, are involved in functions critical to our health and well-being. These bacteria live in our digestive system and play a key role in the digestion of the food we eat, and the absorption and synthesis of nutrients. When the stomach and small intestine are not able to digest certain foods, gut microbes ensure we get the nutrients we need. For instance, whole grains contain non-digestible carbs such as beta-glucan. The small intestine is unable to absorb these carbs, and these make their way to the large intestine, where they are broken down by gut microbes.

From birth until old age, our gut bacteria are constantly evolving. Two-thirds of the gut microbiome is unique to each person. It depends on the food we eat, the air we breathe and other environmental factors. Even identical twins have a different gut microbiome. It also depends on how we arrived in this world. Babies born vaginally have a different type of gut microbiome than those born from caesarean deliveries. Scientists have discovered that while vaginally born babies get most of their gut bacteria from their mother, caesarean babies tend to have more bacteria associated with hospital environments. A number of recent studies have confirmed that babies born via C-sections on average have a less diverse microbe community.[4] It takes longer for them to acquire good strains of bacteria and they also tend to have higher levels of more harmful ones. This lack of microbial diversity is linked to more allergies and respiratory infections.

---

[4]   Josef Neu and Jona Rushing, 'Cesarean versus Vaginal Delivery: Long Term Infant Outcomes and the Hygiene Hypothesis', National Library of Medicine, 2011, https://www.ncbi.nlm.nih.gov/pmc/articles/PMC3110651/ (accessed on 30 July 2020).

Healthy people have a diverse collection of mircroorganisms in their bodies. Most of them are bacteria, but there are viruses, fungi and other microbes as well. In an unhealthy person, however, there is more bacteria associated with different diseases. Such people are more prone to poor immunity, asthma and allergies, obesity, diabetes, heart disease and gut-related conditions, such as irritable bowel syndrome and inflammatory bowel disease. In fact, studies on mice and evidence from human patients show that the microbes in our gut could have a beneficial effect on how well we respond to cancer treatments as well. Antibiotic treatments on melanoma patients have a negative impact on survival rates.[5] Looking after your gut microbiome is as important as looking after your teeth.

Having a less diverse microbiome can lead to absorption of fewer calories from food, the inability to absorb essential minerals and a higher risk of infectious diseases. Diets in a region depend on the ingredients available there. As a result, the microbiomes in the people living in that area adapt to the food and the eating habits of that particular region. The similarities in microbiomes are passed on genetically. For example, people in north India tend to eat more wheat while people in south India eat more rice. The diversity in our microbiomes is the reason no one diet can suit everyone. For example, the Mediterranean diet, which is generally considered excellent, may not suit your gut. To pick the food ideal for your microbiome, you can't just look at how

---

[5]   Weidong Ma et al, 'Gut Microbiota Shapes the Efficiency of Cancer Therapy', National Library of Medicine, 2019, https://www.ncbi. nlm.nih.gov/pmc/articles/PMC6604670/ (accessed on 30 July 2020).

your ancestors ate, as you may now live in a different city or be of mixed heritage. Or it could just be that the same variety of ingredients are not available any more. You need to know what kind of food suits you. Feel free to try out new cuisines and dishes, but avoid foods that cause you discomfort or indigestion. New spices and ingredients can introduce a whole world of benefits.

How a Healthy Gut Turns Unhealthy

It's pretty easy to turn a healthy gut into an unhealthy one. A few bad habits can change the composition of your gut microbiome. I'm listing out some of the most common ones that are really harmful for your gut bacteria:

- *Not eating a variety of foods:* A lack of diversity in gut bacteria limits recovery from infections and from the side-effects of antibiotics. A diet consisting of a wide range of whole foods, such as fruits, vegetables and whole grains, can lead to a more diverse gut flora. In fact, changing your diet from time to time can alter your gut flora profile in just a few days. Foods that have a lot of pesticides, herbicides and fungicides are also bad for the gut microbiome. So find out where and how the food you are consuming has been grown so you know you're eating clean food.
- *Lack of prebiotics in diet:* Prebiotics are fibres that pass through the body undigested and promote the growth and activity of friendly gut bacteria. Many fruits, vegetables and whole grains, such as lentils, chickpeas, bananas, garlic and onions naturally

contain prebiotic fibre. Not enough of this kind of food in your diet is likely to result in poor digestive health.

- *Too much alcohol:* Chronic consumption of alcohol can cause serious problems, such as dysbiosis, which is a form of digestive disturbance. A study examined the gut flora of forty-one alcoholics and compared them to that of ten healthy individuals who consumed little to no alcohol. Twenty-seven per cent of the alcoholic group was seen to have dysbiosis, but not even one in the other group.[6] We'll discuss dysbiosis in detail a little later in this chapter.

- *Abusing antibiotics:* One of the main drawbacks of having antibiotics is that they affect both good and bad bacteria in our bodies. Having antibiotics can lead to long-term alterations in the gut microbiome. After completing a dose of antibiotics, most bacteria return after one to four weeks, but their numbers often don't return to previous levels. In fact, one study found that a single dose of antibiotics reduced the diversity of bacteroides, one of the most dominant bacterial groups in the body, and increased the number of resistant strains. These effects remained for up to two years. Try to first heal your body of infections naturally instead of popping pills indiscriminately.

---

[6] Ece A. Mutlu et al, 'Colonic Microbiome Is Altered in Alcoholism', *American Journal of Physiology*, 2012, https://www.ncbi.nlm.nih.gov/pmc/articles/PMC3362077/ (accessed on 30 July 2020).

If some or all of these habits are part of your lifestyle, it's time to change them. Here is what you can do to bring your gut health back on track.

- *Drink water:* Drink as much water as you can as soon as you wake up. Water helps break down food and move it through the digestive tract. Start with two glasses of water first thing in the morning and keep sipping regularly throughout the day, making sure you have a glass every couple of hours. Water promotes the balance of good bacteria in the gut.

- *Have coffee:* Coffee can dehydrate the body, but when you make sure you stay hydrated, the benefits of coffee are plenty. It has healthy acids, such as chlorogenic acid, and polyphenols. These are antioxidant compounds that have prebiotic properties and hence feed the good bacteria in your gut. The issue with coffee is most often not the coffee—it's what we add to it. That is why black coffee is the best option to maximize benefits from it. At the detox centre in the Philippines, I was given a coffee infusion enema for my colon, also known as the large intestine. The coffee in the enema travelled through the smooth muscle of the small intestine and into the liver. I was told that all of us have built-up layers of colon debris in the form of old mucus deposits and biofilm, which are bacterial overgrowths embedded in the colon walls. The coffee in the enema helps release that debris and overgrowth.

- *Opt for a plant-based diet:* Another excellent way to improve your gut health is to include more plant-based food in your diet. In 2018, the American Society for Microbiology asked 11,000 people about their eating habits and checked their gut microbes. They found that people who had the healthiest guts were those who ate more than thirty types of plants in a week.[7] Plants don't just means vegetables—they can be nuts, seeds, grains, herbs or spices. So if, for instance, you eat butter made from nuts and whole-grain bread for breakfast, a salad at lunch and some cauliflower pizza for dinner, you've eaten a variety of nearly a dozen plants in less than twenty-four hours. All plants in their unrefined forms are high in fibre, which eases digestion.

- *Exercise:* This is my favourite pastime. Isn't it incredible how something that has nothing to do with our diet, nothing to do with what we put into our mouths, can actually change our gut microbiome? Exercise increases the number of good gut microbes, which extract the nutrients in our food and nourish our body. In fact, a 2014 study on Irish rugby players showed that exercise increased microbial diversity in humans.[8] There are a couple of theories on how this works. We don't conclusively know how, but some researchers believe that exercise may impact the integrity of the

---

[7] Daniel McDonald et al, 'American Gut: An Open Platform for Citizen Science Microbiome Research', *mSystems*, 2018, https://msystems.asm.org/content/3/3/e00031-18/figures-only (accessed on 30 July 2020).

[8] S.F. Clarke et al, 'Exercise and Associated Dietary Extremes Impact on Gut Microbial Diversity', *Gut*, 2014, https://gut.bmj.com/content/63/12/1913 (accessed on 30 July 2020).

mucus layer lining of the gut, which supports the growth of beneficial bacteria. Another possibility is that exercises may favourably alter the circulation of bile acids.

- *Check when you eat:* Eating meals at the correct time is extremely important. By cutting out late-night snacking, you give your gut a break. Follow an eating schedule that aligns with the rising and setting of the sun. I eat my dinner by 7 p.m. and after that only drink water till I go to bed. This simple habit has worked wonders for my digestion. Also, chew your food as slowly as you can. Chewing helps break down food and mix it with the saliva, which has enzymes to help break down carbohydrates. When we don't chew our food and mostly swallow it, the gut has to work harder to digest it. So why not come to your stomach's rescue and make its job a little easier?

- *Brush right:* Multiple studies have found that harmful forms of bacteria that grow in the mouth often make their way into the gut. That is why you should brush your teeth well, at least twice a day and particularly after big meals. Floss every day before you hit the bed and visit your dentist at least once every six months.

- *Stay away from sugar:* Other than its ill-effects on our health, sugar also changes the gut microbiome, increasing the amount of bad bacteria in the gut and killing off the good ones. Too much bad bacteria in the gut can lead to inflammation, uneasiness, acne and other health issues. It can even impair the hippocampus, the part of the brain that's associated with memory and emotions. The harmful changes caused to the microbiota by a diet high in processed sugar and fats also extend to the intestine, where the gut microbes live. The walls of the small intestine are meant to keep microorganisms from entering the bloodstream. If they become weak, microorganisms leak into the bloodstream and cause inflammation and other damage. That is why it is best to keep away from food that contains saturated fat, refined sugars or artificial sweeteners.

- *See if your poop floats:* This is an interesting and true fact I learnt from a gastroenterologist. If your poop floats, it could be a sign that there's too much fat in your diet and your intestines may be damaged.
- *Maintain low surround sound:* The sounds you hear before, during and after a meal affect how well your body processes food. The vagus nerve in the body directly connects the brain to the gut. Research has shown that alarming noises can cause digestive spasms, which is why it makes sense to keep your eating environment calm to help your body digest food easier.
- *Walk barefoot:* I make it a point to walk barefoot at home, in the garden, on the sand at the beach and every time I am in the midst of nature. That's how I collect the good bacteria from nature.

Along with these healthy habits, you should also consume foods and spices that are known to do your gut good. I'm listing some of these here:

- *Fermented foods:* Eating fermented foods is the easiest way to introduce beneficial probiotic bacteria to your system. Probiotics are beneficial bacteria, while prebiotics are food for these bacteria. Foods such as kombucha, yoghurt, pickle, kimchi, idli, dosa, sourdough bread and raw cheese (not processed) improve digestion, boost immunity, help treat irritable bowel disease and kill harmful yeast and microbes.

- *Bone broth:* Bone broth is one of my favourite foods to eat. Chicken bone broth contains amino acids such as glycine and glutamine, which keep the gut working well and, hence, help the digestive system run more efficiently. Bone broth has a high concentration of the amino acid glutamine, which improves the function of the intestinal barrier and the structure of its cells. It is also high in the amino acid glycine, which improves antioxidant levels and boosts the mucus layer that protects the lining of the gut.

- *High-fibre fruits:* Whole fruits are usually high in fibre, especially raspberries, pears and apples. Make sure you have pears and apples with their skin on, so you consume all the good fibre. Fibre aids good bowel movement and ensures you poop well. However, make sure you have fruits whole and not juice them, as a lot of the fibre is lost in the process. Mangoes, bananas, pineapples and pomegranates are great.

- *And some more fibre:* We know that our gut microbes thrive when they are fed prebiotic fibre from food, such as yoghurt, sourdough bread and sour pickles. The fibre passes through the small intestine before it reaches the colon. This sets the healthy microbes into a feeding frenzy. They feast on this delicious meal and reward you by releasing short-chain fatty acids. These short-chain fatty acids can help combat a leaky gut, strengthen the immune system, lower cholesterol, prevent diabetes and protect against colon cancer.

- *Chia seeds:* They are full of dietary fibre. Just 100 grams of chia seeds have around 40 grams of dietary fibre, which does wonders for digestion. I have been having chia seeds for years now and recommend this to everyone. Soak them in water for one hour before consuming them.

- *Cayenne pepper:* Cayenne pepper stimulates hydrochloric acid secretion in the stomach, channel pancreatic enzymes into the small intestine and promotes bile secretion in the liver. All three chemicals help digestion and help you feel less bloated after meals. I'd suggest adding some lemon to the pepper for additional gut-boosting benefits.

- *Ginger:* The good ol' Indian spice is great for gut health because it can promote motility through the digestive tract, helping you avoid constipation and bloating. It also works to relieve gut irritation.

- *Oats:* Oatmeal or porridge is rich in a prebiotic fibre called beta glucan, which has been shown to strengthen the immune system. You can add spices and gut-healthy toppings to it as well, such as berries, strawberries and peaches. Just make sure you avoid adding sugar.

- *Apples:* They are a good source of a prebiotic fibre called pectin, which is released from apple skins when heated. Pectin also provides something for your good gut bacteria to feast on. When our bacteria are well fed, they produce short-chain fatty acids, which our gut cells use as fuel.

- *Dark chocolate:* Dark chocolate that has over 75 per cent cocoa is a rich source of polyphenols, which our gut microbes love and thrive on.
- *Cumin seeds:* Cumin can help bile production, which is what your body needs to break down fat, so that it can be digested and absorbed. When your body has a hard time breaking down fat, you feel sluggish and bloated. Munch on a few cumin seeds after a rich meal to stay energized.
- *Fennel seeds:* Fennel seeds promote a healthy gut by fighting the bad bacteria that can build up in the gut and cause indigestion and discomfort. I incorporate them into my diet by sprinkling some on top of my stir-fries and soups.
- *Turmeric:* Turmeric is a natural laxative. While it is part of most Indian food, I also have turmeric tablets to boost my gut health. Turmeric contains a phytochemical called curcumin, which has some extraordinary healing properties. It also protects the liver and suppresses cancer cells. You can also slice a turmeric pod, dip it in lemon for a few days and have it as a pickle.
- *Kimchi:* Kimchi is made from fermented vegetables and is packed with fibre, and vitamins A and C.
- *Broccoli:* One of my favourite veggies, broccoli is great for gut health. It releases a phytochemical called sulforaphane, which heals the gut and reduces inflammation.
- *Smoothies:* Smoothies are a great way to add a mix of fruits and vegetables to your diet. The best way

to get a healthy gut microbiome is to have diverse plants in your diet. Add banana and greens in your smoothies, along with ground flax, chia and hemp seeds, and walnuts or almonds for fibre.

Research shows that your response to food is initially determined by the microorganisms that inhabit your gut.[9] So if you lack certain fibre-eating microbes, this will affect your ability to process fibre, and it may be a while before these microbes grow and prosper in your gut. So eating fibre-rich foods such as whole grains, apples and broccoli will speed up the process.

The Leaky Gut Syndrome

Approximately 2,000 different strains of bacteria live inside or on us. In fact, it is estimated that bacterial cells outnumber human cells in the body. However, not all bacteria in the gut are beneficial—too many undesirable strains of bacteria can take a major toll on our immunity.

When bad bacteria outnumber the good, it is called dysbiosis. Over time, this can lead to a leaky gut. This means the intestinal lining no longer functions efficiently as a barrier to keep microorganisms out of the bloodstream. This may cause the immune system to constantly be on high alert and lead to inflammation. This is also well documented in Ayurveda. Ama is an undigested product derived from

---

[9] Michael A. Conlon and Anthony R. Bird, 'The Impact of Diet and Lifestyle on Gut Microbiota and Human Health', *Nutrients*, 2014, https://www.ncbi.nlm.nih.gov/pmc/articles/PMC4303825/ (accessed on 30 July 2020).

food that gets absorbed into the system without proper assimilation. Such partly digested material is of no use to the system and acts to clog the body, which brings about an immune reaction. A few things you can do to fix a leaky gut are:

- Remove inflammatory foods.
- Consider supplements such as aloe, glutamine, licorice and L-carnitine.
- Add probiotics to help populate the gut with good bacteria.

If you experience frequent gastrointestinal discomfort, your body is trying to send you a message. Listen to it. It is wise to remove inflammatory foods such as sugar, trans fat and refined flour from your diet and add anti-inflammatory foods to it. These include green tea; herbs and spices such as basil, cinnamon, curry powder, garlic, ginger, rosemary, thyme and turmeric; legumes such as lentils and chickpeas; edamame; soya milk; nuts and seeds such as almonds, chia, flax and walnuts; grains such as basmati rice, quinoa, barley and brown rice; vegetables such as beets, carrots, broccoli, cabbage, cauliflower, kale, spinach, onions and peas; shiitake mushrooms; and fruits such as apples, blackberries, blueberries, cherries, oranges, peaches, pears, plums, pomegranates, raspberries and strawberries.

Food is not just calories—it is information. The body is made up of cells and nerves. When you feed it something bad, your body reacts badly to it, giving you inflammation and making you feel sluggish. The quality of the food you eat plays a huge role in your ability to digest it.

If you regularly experience indigestion, bloating or discomfort, you have to check whether you are stressed more than usual. I know that I return to the topic of stress again and again, but it's because everything in our bodies is connected and what happens in one part affects the other. Ninety per cent of the feel-good hormone serotonin that the brain releases is produced in the gut. Stress to the system impacts the whole body. Stress often leads to bad food choices. How often have you reached for some junk food when you've had a bad, stressful day? We are all guilty of that. Reaching for a burger instead of vegetables is all right once in a while. But doing this repeatedly just isn't good for you. Stress also leads to poor sleep habits, which lead to internal stress. When we eat things such as fried food, white flour and sugar, we increase inflammation and the production of stress hormones.

If you're already suffering from a leaky gut, it's important to take care of your diet so you can slowly get better and heal your gut. Here are a few foods you should eat:

Protein: Organic chicken, grass-fed beef, lamb and organic or free-range eggs

Carbohydrates: Porridge oats, brown rice, brown rice pasta and brown rice noodles

Fats: Avocado, all nuts except peanuts, almond butter or any nut butter other than peanut butter, olive oil and rapeseed oil

Vegetables: Everything green is great—cucumber, celery, lettuce, spinach, kale, sprouts, peas and broad beans. Peppers, aubergine, cabbage, broccoli, etc., can be eaten in large amounts. Avoid root vegetables such as potato, sweet potato and carrots.

Pulses: Chickpeas, kidney beans, lentils and quinoa are all good.

It's just as important to stay away from foods that will make your condition worse. These are:

Sugars: Sugar, honey syrup, chocolate and artificial sweeteners tend to be high in sugar. Stay away from soft drinks too. Always read food labels to make sure your food doesn't contain sugar. This goes for artificial sweeteners as well. Aspartame in diet cola weakens your immune system.

Alcohol: Drinking a lot of alcohol can lead to a temporary drop in your blood sugar, but moderate amounts tend to increase it. Alcoholic drinks are often full of carbohydrates and have high sugar mixers and foods. In the long run, alcohol consumption tends to decrease the effectiveness of insulin, leading to consistently higher blood-sugar levels. Alcohol can also increase gut permeability and negatively affect your immune system.

Meats: All pork products, cured meats, processed meats, smoked or vacuum-packed meats. Pork contains retroviruses that survive cooking and may be harmful for those with a weak digestive system.

Dairy products: All dairy, such as milk, butter, cheese, yoghurt, cream and whey products should be avoided. Milk contains lactose, a sugar, which is not good for someone with a leaky gut.

Additives and preservatives: Manufactured citric acid is derived from yeast. However, the natural form, as found in lemons and limes, is okay in the diet. Additives and preservatives will disrupt and kill the good bacteria in your gut. If you don't know what an ingredient is, or can't pronounce it, don't eat it.

Condiments: Ketchup, tomato paste, spaghetti sauces, mustard, mayonnaise and soya sauce all contain high amounts of hidden sugars. For an alternative salad dressing, try simple olive oil and lemon juice.

Fruits: While fruits are great for most people, if you are suffering from a leaky gut, stay away from them because they all contain sugar, even though natural.

The Healthy Gut Pyramid

I believe Oprah Winfrey is one of the smartest women in the world. When she endorsed the psychobiotic food pyramid, I knew we all had to pay attention to what she was saying. The model was created by John Cryan and Ted Dinan, from the University of Cork, who co-authored the book *The Psychobiotic Revolution*. It's a simple approach to the sometimes-complicated topic of eating a gut-healthy diet.

The pyramid has four layers. The food mentioned at the bottom has to be eaten abundantly and on a regular basis. As you go up the pyramid, the food quantity reduces and the interval of eating increases.

The base layer is made up of vegetables, fruits, whole grains, legumes, olive oil, herbs and spices. They are to be eaten daily. Layer 2 is made up of fish, seafood and fermented food. They should be eaten often. Layer 3 has poultry, eggs and dairy, which should be consumed once a week. Finally, the top layer has red meat and sweets, and should be eaten rarely.

The creators of the psychobiotic food pyramid say that reducing the foods you eat from layers 3 and 4 is more important than increasing the nutrients of layers 1 and 2. However, this is a generalized pyramid and may not be applicable to everyone, especially if you have underlying conditions. So be mindful when you follow it and always listen to your body.

How I Bettered My Gut

The tips I've spoken about till now are general guidelines, but we must not forget that our bodies are unique and demand specific care. Your gut, too, needs special attention because what irritates your gut may not irritate someone else's. Overall, gluten, dairy, corn, eggs, yeast and soya are the most common gut irritants. If you have been facing bowel issues, you need to find out which of these six irritants is bothering you. The best way to do this is to eat food from only one of the groups at a time: gluten, dairy, corn, eggs, yeast or soya for two or three days, along with vegetables, fruits and nuts. Try out one food group at a time until you've seen how you digest each of them. Observe how your body reacts to all of them. Does your mood change? Do your joints feel sore? Does your tummy feel odd? If the answer is yes, you know it's affecting your gut adversely. When in doubt, leave it out.

It's important to make sure you avoid the other groups while having a particular food group. If you've had a migraine on the day you ate corn and had a glass of milk, you won't know what caused the reaction. If you have symptoms, wait till they abate—give it three days—before trying the next irritant. Continue this until you have tested all the six irritants. It was through this process that I discovered my intolerance to lactose.

I got my gut to work at its optimum best by clearing it completely. I began by drinking my green juice and a lot of water throughout the day. You can find the greens I add to my special concoction in the chapter on diet. I also ate fruits with high fibre, such as apples, bananas, oranges and strawberries. Activated charcoal pills did a fantastic job to clear my gut and remove inflammation. Activated charcoal is a fine, odourless, black powder. The powder stops toxins from being absorbed in the stomach by binding to them, thus reducing inflammation and giving you a clean gut. Consuming bread, ice cream, yoghurt and pizza made from activated charcoal had become a fad a few years ago. But I did some research and found out that activated charcoal is supposed to be had on an empty stomach because it attaches to the toxins in your body and flushes it out. When people have activated charcoal with food, it gets attached to all the important nutrients and flushes them out. You definitely don't want that to happen. I take a probiotic supplement and prebiotic foods such as kombucha, high-fibre foods and kimchi to enhance good bacteria in my gut.

Alkalizing my body by eating sweet potato, yam, slow-cooked brown rice and seaweed also helped. When the body is in an alkaline state, you are less likely to suffer from chronic disease and illness. My family and I switched to alkaline water a few years ago and it has really made a difference.

Having a balanced pH level in the body is essential for good health and vitality. The body's pH level determines whether its fluids and tissues are more acidic or alkaline.

The scale varies from - 4.5 (which is very acidic) to 9.5 (which is highly alkaline), and the body usually tries to maintain equilibrium at a pH of 7.365, which is slightly alkaline.

My Detox Experience

This chapter would be incomplete if I didn't share my experiences at The Farm at San Benito. I returned from my week there in a completely different state of mind and body. I had heard rave reviews about The Farm and each turned out to be true. It is a wellness centre that is frequented by people around the world. For the detox programme, I chose to focus on my liver, kidney and colon. Making sure they worked at their optimum best was my goal. So I decided to go vegan while I was there. It is the best way to eat whenever you are detoxing. As you know, I do not believe in diets. I believe in nourishing my body with the healthiest food that suits it. While choosing a detox programme, twenty-one days is ideal. You require that time because the body needs three weeks to break any habit. I understand that it is difficult to find this time for ourselves, especially with our hectic lives and responsibilities. But sometimes we have to make our health a priority and give our body the love it needs.

I was accompanied to The Farm by my daughter, who works in Los Angeles. So, along with the benefits of wellness, I also got to spend some time with my best friend and my baby, who I don't see as often as I would like to.

At The Farm, I began the day with a turmeric shot. Haldi is known to work wonders for our liver. It increases the production of vital enzymes that are responsible for detoxifying our blood that goes to the liver by breaking down toxins. That apart, I loved the natural juices they served us every day. They did wonders for my system. I have shared them all below, so you, too, can blend yourself a glass when you need a dose of natural goodness. Just blitz all the ingredients together in a food processor or juicer.

Green Magnet Juice: 89 calories

Ingredients: Romaine lettuce, cucumber and cilantro

Cilantro has an excellent heavy-metal chelating effect that, when consumed, is able to bind with toxic metals and escort them out of the body. It also has antimicrobial properties that are beneficial for the gut. This juice detoxes the body of heavy metals.

Electric Spice Juice: 70 calories

Ingredients: Lettuce, cucumber, parsley and turmeric

This helps the body absorb nutrients from leafy greens more easily than when you chew them. This drink is packed with nutrition and low on the glycemic index. This is also rich in magnesium, calcium, potassium, and vitamins A and C.

Alkaline Booster Juice: 104 calories

Ingredients: Broccoli, lettuce, cucumber, celery, lime juice and moringa

This juice helps your body maintain a slightly alkaline state. It has a unique and powerful ability to aid your body in detoxification. Another benefit is that it has high amounts of antioxidants. Broccoli is full of vitamin B1 and has a generous amount of calcium, sulphur and potassium as well.

Tropical Mint: 115 calories

Ingredients: Lettuce, cucumber, celery and mint
  This aids in cleansing the body, thanks to the presence of bromelain, a powerful digestive enzyme that helps breakdown of fats and reduction of inflammation.

Ginger Beet Detox Juice: 127 calories

Ingredients: Beet, cucumber, celery, cilantro, lime and ginger
  Beets are rich in natural irons and cleanse the blood beautifully. They also have anti-inflammatory properties, and are a good source of calcium and vitamin K to help prevent bone loss. To sharpen and tone the flavour, ginger was added to enhance digestive properties.

Green Lemonade Juice: 84 calories

Ingredients: Cucumber, celery and lime
  Citrus fruits are known for their detoxification properties. The vitamin C content stimulates glutathione production in the liver, which is beneficial for your immune system. This refreshing juice is alkalizing, oxygenating, rich in enzymes, minerals and nutrient, and helps eject waste.

Ginger Zinger: 96 calories

Ingredients: Carrots, celery, ginger and lime
  Citric acid and ginger are wonderful at eliminating toxins, aiding digestion and stimulating metabolism. This juice is rich in vitamin C, which helps sweep off free radicals and keeps tissues strong and healthy.

Food for Thought

Eating well doesn't just benefit your body, it also benefits your brain. So what exactly should you eat to improve your brain health? Foods high in omega-3 fats, vitamin B12, zinc, magnesium and iron, found in whole foods, legumes, lean red meat, fruits, veggies, olive oil and nuts, are all good for your microbiome and, consequently, your brain. While it is possible to have omega-3 fats, vitamin B12, zinc, magnesium and iron as supplements, it is much better to consume them in natural form. As food, they lower inflammation, leading to better gut health.

Oats, lentils, quinoa and beans have also been linked to brain health. All the complex carbohydrates stabilize blood sugar levels because of their fibre and phytonutrient content, which keeps the mood and energy stable in the short term and promotes healthy brain function in the long run. Not all carbs are bad. If you choose lentils, beans and whole grains over refined carbs such as maida and potatoes, your gut and brain both will be happier.

Signs You May Have a Build-Up of Toxicity

- Sugar cravings
- Low or inconsistent energy
- Bloating or gas
- Caffeine addiction
- Binge-eating or drinking
- Mood swings/irritability/anxiety
- Brain fog or difficulty concentrating
- Fluid retention
- Migraines or headaches

Self-Care

While I have concentrated so far on overall health, and gut health in particular, the conversation cannot be complete without talking about mental health. In our fast-paced lives, it is more important than ever to take care of our mental health. For me, the first step to that is self-care.

The World Health Organisation defines self-care as the ability of individuals, families and communities to promote and maintain health, prevent disease and cope with illness with or without the support of a healthcare provider.[10] A simpler version says that you need to pay attention to and support your own physical and mental health.

Many of us have so many responsibilities that we forget to take care of our own needs. Adulthood is hard and sometimes we wish we could have had the carefree days of our childhood back. We have deadlines to meet and so much work to do at home. Add social events and other activities to that, and who wouldn't want to trade places with our younger selves?

So what does self-care mean to you? Is it pampering yourself with regular mani-pedis? Is it getting massages or watching TV all day?

Yes, it can include all of this, but it should also be so much more. Ask yourself what your deepest desire is. Is something holding you back from achieving it? Listening to that voice is self-care. It is about putting yourself first

---

[10] 'Self-Care Can Be an Effective Part of National Health Systems', World Health Organization, 2019, https://www. who.int/reproductivehealth/self-care-national-health-systems/ en/#:~:text=Included%20in%20the%20World%20Health,a%20 health%2Dcare%20provider.%E2%80%9D (accessed on 30 July 2020).

every once in a while, not neglecting yourself and checking in with your state of mind regularly. By taking your own needs and wants into consideration, you maintain a healthy relationship with yourself. A lot of people feel guilty about indulging themselves. They feel that they are being selfish by putting themselves first. I'm sure a lot of women in particular feel this way because we have been brought up in a society that equates a good woman with sacrifice. But that could not be farther from the truth. When you pay adequate attention to your well-being, you're not considering your needs alone—you're refuelling yourself so that you can be the best version of yourself for the people around you as well. Everyone around you also benefits from your renewed joy and energy. A good way to constantly reinforce self-love and self-care is to document the moments you feel most in love with yourself—note what you're wearing, who's around you and what you're doing. Observe what makes you happy, and recreate and repeat these instances as often as possible.

Self-care is more than eating and exercising right. It is much more than just feeling okay. Feeling well means feeling whole, vibrant, balanced and alive. You want to show up in this world as the best and healthiest version of yourself. You can do that by loving yourself wholeheartedly. Fall in love with taking care of yourself, through the path of deep healing, patience, compassion and respect—and trust the process of becoming your truest self.

Self-care comes in many forms. While one aspect is about becoming a better version of yourself, another is about listening to your heart and doing what you feel is right. We are all taught that a person who conquers their fear is brave. But don't forget that it's just as brave to admit to a fear. Doing so makes us vulnerable. By expressing that we are scared of something, we are also putting ourselves first. I have always told my children that it's all right to be scared sometimes. There is no shame in admitting that. In fact, people who do that are probably the bravest people on the planet. For instance, I do not like roller coasters at all, and no one can convince me to go on one. I have no problem admitting it, because I care for myself and don't want to go on an adventure ride at an amusement park just to prove something. It would probably do nothing to alleviate my fear of roller coasters.

Self-care must take into account your physical, mental and spiritual health. Let's think of each of these individually.

Physical health: This includes sleep, massages, diet, exercise, outdoor time and acupuncture. Get regular sleep around the same time every day. That way you will wake up feeling fresh and be ready to take on the day. Regular hour-long massages will help relieve stress and anxiety, and leave your body feeling limber. There is so much I can say about diet, but all I'll mention here is that without feeding yourself healthy, nutritious food, you will never be able to be your best self. The same holds true for exercise. I'd also recommend spending time outdoors every day—preferably in the middle of nature—to reap its many benefits. You will come back home with a clearer mind. Finally, acupuncture is a holistic treatment that takes into account the physical, mental, emotional and spiritual aspects of your health and well-being. It calms your nervous system and definitely reduces stress. If your lifestyle allows it, get a pet. They are great for gut health because they share their microorganisms with you.

Emotional health: This includes laughing, reading, hobbies, travelling and indulging in creative activities. There is a reason why laughter clubs are so popular in India. Laughing without inhibitions and feeling happy while doing so go a long way in reducing any stress you're feeling at that point. Read when you can find the time, during your commute to work or before you go to sleep, because it relaxes your mind and fires up your imagination. Also, pursue a hobby. It could be anything you enjoy doing—whether it's playing an instrument, crocheting, exercising or cooking. It will give you a break from your routine and keep burnout at bay. The benefits of travelling, of course, are well known. A change of scenery and leaving your troubles back home can do wonders for your spirit and recharge you to face your day-to-day routine when you are back home.

Spiritual health: Forgive. By doing so, you will begin the process of healing and be free of the emotions that may be holding you back. It is also wise to forgive yourself for any transgression you think you may have done. You are a flawed person, just like everyone else, and you need to give yourself a break when you are being too harsh on yourself. Be gentle and kind with yourself. It is also important to meditate. The chapter on spirituality will tell you more about why it is probably the best gift you can give yourself, as well as how to do it. Also, be grateful for all that you have and all that you have achieved. It will make you feel like everything is right with the world. Believe that you have enough and that you are enough.

Relationship with Yourself

You can begin to have a better relationship with yourself by identifying the things that matter to you the most. Ask yourself:

- When things aren't going well, who do you want to be with?
- How do you want others to know and remember you?
- How do you want to make a difference in the world?

Your answers will help you determine your approach to living. Spend more time with those you love to be with and live your life in a way that people remember you the way you want them to. Celebrate all your successes, no matter how small, because you matter.

At Work

Our career is what gives most of us our identity. That's how other people know us. Even while we're climbing the ladder of success, there are some self-care rules that apply at office too. Make sure to set boundaries so no one takes advantage of your good nature; say no when you want to; take time off whenever you are overwhelmed and need a break; set goals to maximize your potential; learn new skills; support and acknowledge yourself and the others you work with; and advocate for yourself when the need arises.

Relationship with Others

Spend time with family, friends and children—you will know how loved and cherished you are. You can also get involved with a cause and spend a few hours a week helping others with their lives.

Being the CEO of your body and life is the best thing you can do for yourself.

Make all these aspects of self-care regular parts of your routine, not just something you do occasionally. Call up someone close to you. Fit in time for movement. Cook a meal. Set up daily or monthly affirmations. Take an inventory of what makes you happy. Incorporate meditation into your daily routine. All these aspects are very personal and individual. Treat yourself as you would a child—with respect, honesty and undivided attention.

Final Thoughts

Your involvement in your own self-care will ebb and flow. The areas of your life that need balance will shift, and the ways you want to fill those needs will change as well. How self-care looks in your life may change drastically from one period to the next, but it's important that you make a consistent effort in caring for yourself. The art of self-love is a lifelong practice, so be easy on yourself and take it one day at a time. Here are a few things you can do:

- Take time each week to check in with yourself and identify the areas you need support in.
- Choose the activities you would like to engage in on a weekly basis.
- Schedule time in your calendar for each activity.
- Enlist the support of friends and family to make those activities a success.
- Trust people you care for to take care of themselves, so that you can take care of yourself.
- Be present and mindful during self-care rituals.

Keep Your Gut Healthy while Travelling

- *Stick to your routine:* A friend of mine eats nuts and seeds every morning. She carries pistachios, walnuts, almonds and sunflower seeds in a small bag whenever she travels. What makes you feel your best in your day-to-day life is just as essential on vacation.

- *Carry water:* Dehydration is the cause of many issues—constipation, low energy, headaches, cramps and sugar cravings. Carry a bottle of water with you. It'll also be better for the planet than buying single-use plastic bottles when you feel thirsty.

- *Pack probiotics:* This will help you keep your digestion smooth. Have kombucha and yoghurt while travelling.

- *Plan your diet:* Pack a bag with snacks to avoid frozen food at airports and on flights. For the flight, pack cooked greens, roasted veggies and avocado.

- *Practise post-plane yoga:* Be sure to stretch frequently. It will help your ligaments and muscles, and also aid movement in your stomach and gut.

- *Eat your greens:* Consuming a plate of vegetables a day along with proteins, carbohydrates and healthy fats will ensure a healthy gut during your travels.

- *Take digestive enzymes:* On days you're enjoying exotic cuisines your body isn't used to, it needs a little more help to digest the food. Digestive enzymes help your body break down carbs, proteins and fats, and utilize them to reduce bloating and relieve digestive issues. If you find them expensive, have some papaya or pineapple after every meal.

- *Try intermittent fasting:* Travelling across time zones can cause your system to slow down. In that case, intermittent fasting helps to increase energy and circulation, gives your detoxifying organs support and stabilizes your metabolism. If you are travelling at night, spend the day eating food that is easy to digest and give the airplane food a miss. Once you land, have your next meal at the same time as the local eating time.

PHYSICAL WELLNESS

Too fit to quit.

Four months into the pandemic, I had a chance to go to Alibag with some friends. I'm grateful to have been comfortable and happy at home during those months and was missing only one thing—being outdoors, in the midst of nature. As you'll read in more detail in the next chapter, appreciating nature's beauty is a way for me to connect deeply with my inner self. It's a balm for my soul and helps me be one with my surroundings and the world, a way to stand still and take a slow, deep breath amid the constant motion of life. When my friends, with whom I had created a social bubble (where we only met each other), asked me to come along, I thought it would be the perfect way to rejuvenate that side of me.

The day of the journey I woke up with slight acidity and a headache. I had eaten a home-cooked meal for dinner—nothing that should have caused the discomfort. It was probably my body telling me that it was time to do a mini detox and go back to nature. I thought the headache and acidity would eventually go away, and so stuck to my routine and had a healthy breakfast of idli with a couple of fruits.

On the journey there, the headache got worse, but I tried to focus on my breathing and calming my mind, hoping my body would follow suit. I didn't want to take medicines, because I don't believe in rushing to just manage a symptom. After so many years of tuning in to my body and understanding what works for it, I kept the faith that I would soon feel better.

When we reached and got down from the car, I couldn't help but spread my arms wide and close my eyes. With a smile on my face, I breathed in the clean, fresh air. I smiled at the lush field in front of me, with hardly anyone else in sight. Tall trees swayed gently in the breeze, as though calling out. I felt a deep sense of calm, and it allowed me to take my mind off the discomfort I was feeling in my body.

As soon as I could, I set off on the trail around the property, barefoot. I wanted to connect with the earth, feel it under my feet, be one with it. Walking through the grass, with an overcast sky, I felt so alive. It felt like part of me had been asleep and was waking up in the breeze that blew in from the sea. I soon reached a grove of trees—tall, sturdy casuarinas rising up to meet the open sky. I slowly walked amid them, drinking in all the beauty, letting the sights and sounds of nature nourish me. This is wellness to me, above everything else. Something that connects to an integral part of me, touches me deeply and leaves me feeling like a whole new person. It's not just about going to the gym and burning a certain number of calories. It's about expanding the mind, finding the connection with my surroundings, absorbing the right energy my body needs and letting it exist in the most natural way it is supposed to.

Beyond the trees was the beach, with no one to see the waves gently break on the sand except me. I walked along the water, letting the waves wash my feet, and felt the grains of sand beneath me. I took it all in and felt part of something so much larger than myself, but also how I was an integral, living, breathing part of it. At the end of the beach, when it was time to turn around, I realized that my stomach was so much better and my headache was nearly gone. Without even putting any extra thought or effort into it, I had walked for forty minutes, focused on myself and lived in the present. And it had done wonders for me.

And this is how I define physical wellness. Physical wellness is not just following a regimen or workout because you're supposed to. It's about understanding your body, enjoying time with yourself and experiencing the true joy that comes from being active. This is why even after thirty-five years of working out, I look forward to it every day, eager to get started. When I'm not in the mood to go to the gym, I pick up something else instead, something that speaks to me and what my body needs. It could be a run in the park, some yoga or even a lovely long walk in the forest.

Wellness and fitness mean different things to different people. But they both begin with making choices towards a healthy and fulfilling life. Wellness is more than just being free of illness. It is a process of change and growth, and includes taking care of your physical appearance as well as emotional well-being. It's a lifelong journey, during which you constantly work to take care of yourself. Wellness is important, because everything we do and every emotion we feel relates to our well-being. In turn, our well-being affects our actions and emotions.

Open a fashion magazine and you'll see people who look like the picture of good health. Their bodies are slim and toned. Their stomachs are flat. They look confident. We look at them and think they look perfect. But perfection is a dangerous goal for fitness. No one starts out as an amazing athlete or in peak shape. It takes time, focus and hard work. Also, fitness is not just about looking slim. There's so much more to fitness than just being the right weight or being able to fit into clothes of a particular size. Unless you feel strong and energetic, eat well and exercise in a way that doesn't harm you in the long run, you are not fit. In this chapter, I'm not going to prescribe exact exercises, along with a fixed number of reps and sets that you must do. That's because fitness is as individual as you are. You're a unique person, so you have to understand and learn what works for you on a regular basis, what your goals are and what your current state is physically and emotionally, and then decide on the kind of physical activity you want to maintain and improve your fitness. I can vouch for the fact that there is no better feeling than being fit. You don't need a perfect body or run a marathon to feel this way. All you have to do is not settle for less than the best for you.

It is more important to determine what you want to be able to do, i.e., to set a goal for yourself. For some, it could be to compete in a marathon. For others, it could be the ability to play with their children without getting tired. Consider your abilities as well as your limitations. Once you do this, you'll actively put your mind and body in the best possible state to achieve that goal. It'll become easier to adjust your diet, exercises and schedule, as you're working towards something you truly want. Remember that all of us are capable of doing more than we think. But if you never try, you'll never know what you can achieve.

The What of It

All activities can be categorized as strength, cardiovascular, flexibility, mobility and balance training. Rest and recovery is also part of physical fitness. I find that rest and recovery is often not considered part of fitness, but that is a wrong approach, as it's rest—both active and passive—that allows your body to soak up all the benefits of exercise and make sure you can keep doing it for a longer period of time without injury. Strength training involves activities where you're working particular muscle groups; cardio is anything that gets the heart pumping and makes you do active work; flexibility increases the length of the muscles; mobility improves the range of motion of each joint; and balance exercises help improve stability. It's important that you work in different types of exercises into your fitness routine. For example, if you're focusing on improving stamina but don't build enough muscle mass, you leave yourself more prone to injury. To work in all these components of exercises, you can pick two or three different activities to do throughout the week. For example, choose zumba, which is a great form of cardio and can improve mobility, for a couple of days, and do calisthenics or lift weights for two days a week. Another day in the week can be kept for yoga, and possibly two days that are just for resting. For exact guidance on which exercise to do for each kind of activity, along with suggested reps and sets, you can turn to my book, *Shut Up and Train!*.

Walking, running, push-ups, pull-ups, squats and lunges are the most basic movements and extremely important for the body. Make sure these are part of your fitness routine, no matter what activity you pick.

Sometimes, the stress of just getting through each day can make you tired of working out. That's because exercise in itself is a stressor. An intense workout or one involving heavier weights causes micro-tears in your muscles. When the body recovers, your immune system works to repair those tears, making your muscles stronger than they were before. So stress in a small amount is good. The problem begins when that stress becomes too much. You should come home from a workout physically drained and mentally refreshed. If you feel drained both mentally and physically—as is known to happen in the hurried times we live in—you're probably overstressing your body. A study has found that prolonged mental stress increases the amount of fatigue and soreness by up to four days post-workout.[1]

That is why in times of stress and crisis, don't turn to just heavy-duty and strenuous stuff, like an HIIT or a CrossFit session. Make sure you also do yoga, because it builds you up physically and calms the mind. Coupled with meditation, it helps to slow you down. For example, during the pandemic, when I could not go to the gym, I chose to increase the number of days I focused on yoga. I went inwards—body, mind and soul. It felt right for me, because it is more calming and helps keep anxiety at bay. Sure, I was losing muscle mass—I even had flab around the arms and stomach—but that didn't bother me at all, because I knew that when I started going to the gym, it would all go away. If you don't know where to begin, the basic surya namaskar is a full-body workout and very good for you. Start with ten to fifteen and work your way up. The number of repetitions

---

[1] Stults-Kolehmainen et al, 'Chronic Psychological Stress Impairs Recovery of Muscular Function and Somatic Sensations Over a 96-Hour Period', *Journal of Strength and Conditioning Research*, 2014, https://journals.lww.com/nsca-jscr/Fulltext/2014/07000/Chronic_Psychological_Stress_Impairs_Recovery_of.26.aspx (accessed on 17 August 2020).

is something you need to decide. My mantra is that you should keep going a little beyond the point at which you feel comfortable. You can also turn to exercises such as cycling and swimming, which are both good for the joints, in case you don't do yoga.

I don't recommend strenuous workouts when you're going through a mentally challenging time, because it's easy to think that you can hit the gym with a vengeance and channel anger, grief and frustration into your workout. But you may end up injuring yourself or quickly lose the will to exercise. When you are stressed or angry, the body gets into fight-or-flight mode, releasing cortisol. So a stressful workout will add to it. In such times, give your body some love and stretch, foam-roll or do an easy cardio or strength-training session. If you're a runner, go for a walk. If you love spin classes, go for a relaxing bike ride. It's a myth that you always have to do something rigorous for it to count as exercise. It should be whatever you are in the mood for that day. You can do water aerobics, pool yoga or even an animal walk, such as a bear crawl, lizard walk, frog leap or monkey walk. These replicate the movements of these animals and will help you stretch and strengthen your muscles in a different and highly effective way.

On days you do have energy and are in a good space mentally, by all means burn those calories. A good run is one of the best forms of cardio. I'm more inclined to go running on the grass, barefoot, as it feels more natural to me, but you can always run on a treadmill or even tackle the cross trainer or upper-body rower to get your heart pumping. Other excellent options are HIIT, which will incorporate body-weight exercises and work in a lot of the basic movements we discussed—squats, lunges, push-ups, pull-ups—in quick succession and with short bursts of power. Similarly, CrossFit, weight-training, boot camp, spin classes, stationary bikes are good for high-energy workouts.

There's one major mistake that many of us make while doing HIIT—we push ourselves too hard. We should go all out during our exercises but then rest if we have to recover fully. But if we aren't giving ourselves enough time to recover, our workout won't be as effective. If we are operating at 100 per cent throughout the workout, we are likely getting some great endurance training, but we will be missing out on the metabolism boost after HIIT. So how do we know we are doing it right? We should become 'breathless' multiple times during the workout, so we know we are reaching our greatest intensity level. And from there, we need to slow down and rest.

Keep in mind your surroundings. If you live in a hot and humid place such as Mumbai, don't do hot yoga or run in the humid summers at noon, as it will drain your energy. Similarly, when you travel, you might find your food habits altered because of the weather. Even if you're coming from a hot country, you might crave soup in a cold country or wholesome grains in humid weather. Stop for a few minutes, close your eyes and take a few deep breaths. Think of what you are in the mood for and instinctively choose that. You won't go wrong in your choice. When I travel, I like to visit the best parks in that city. That way I also take in a beautiful landmark and spend some time in nature. You could always also plan an adventure sport, a marathon, a trek or a hike, mountain-biking or some fitness classes, as the gyms in other countries often have new and unique programmes.

Rather than struggle with your environment, you should make it work for you. For example, I love training with resistance bands and the TRX. They are lightweight and very versatile. You can attach them to a tree, a pole, a door or anything sturdy, and use them to work the arms, the legs or even as a warm-up. They are particularly prescribed for those who have injuries, as the movements from using a resistance band cushions the joints and helps improve strength. You can use them at the gym, at the park, at home or even in office. The best thing is you can take them along wherever you travel. I took them on my trip to Alibag, put them on a couple of trees and did pull-ups and arm exercises. I always used to think I don't have enough strength to do a pull-up, but a couple of years ago, I started using resistance bands to help me, as they create some momentum and help you pull your body up. Now I've reached the point where I can do a pull-up without a band too. You can even incorporate resistance bands into your HIIT workouts. This is known as high-intensity resistance training (HIRT) and focuses on adding strength-based exercises rather than cardiovascular ones.

There are times when you won't be able to step out of your home for an activity. All of us were homebound for months during the pandemic, unable to follow our usual schedules. For many, this meant they couldn't go the gym or to a class. But this doesn't mean you should give up exercise. Rather, use the things around you to add variation to your fitness regime when at home. I adapted during those months by using the stairs at home. I would first warm up by climbing up and down, till I had climbed for seven or eight floors. This was my cardio. I then did speed drills and then lower-body exercises to work the thighs and hamstrings, which exercised my muscles. The next couple of days I worked on my upper body and core using the stairs. Similarly, I did wall workouts, where I did headstands or wall push-ups, or a couch workout, which was a great way to do tricep dips and squats.

I also did workouts using a backpack, water bottles, socks, hand towels, a chair, a stick and other household items. You can find all these exercises on my Instagram account, @deannepanday.

I recommend that you do something completely different one day of the week. This will wake up the body from the usual workout you gravitate to. For example, when I was at Alibag, I did backward running on the beach. Ideally, to improve mobility and agility, you should move your body in every direction. When we walk backwards, we engage the brain to learn how to do an everyday movement differently. You can do backward running in any empty space, as it'll engage a different group of muscles. Just make sure you don't go too fast, keep your head steady and be aware of your surroundings.

I can't speak of fitness without touching upon weight training. It's been one of the mainstays of my fitness routine and has helped me age well. It's what I feel most comfortable doing and derive the most joy from. There's something so exhilarating about lifting weights in the right posture. For people who want to put more emphasis on strength training, always start with body-weight exercises and then build up to adding more weights. When you no longer feel the burn easily with your own body weight, use kettlebells and dumb-bells. Deadlifts, squats, lunges, push-ups and pull-ups are, of course, basic movements. There are many exercises that build on these movements and help ramp up the difficulty level.

Weight training is extremely beneficial, but one of the risks is lifting weights too heavy or not being able to maintain the right form through the reps. The best way to avoid injury is to do the most number of reps at the beginning of the workout and then keep reducing that number. You're the strongest at the beginning of your workout, when your muscles aren't tired, and it'll help you maintain good form and momentum till the end.

Callisthenics are body-weight exercises, such as squats, lunges and push-ups, which don't require any equipment. Instead of lifting equipment as in the case of weight training, you're lifting the weight of your body. Lifting weights trains specific muscles while callisthenics improve balance, coordination and range of motion. For example, a push-up is a callisthenics exercise that works the chest, the triceps, the shoulders and the core, but a chest press works just the chest. It's best to do both types of exercises. Callisthenics and weight training go together, so you can derive the maximum benefit from both.

I would also recommend doing inversion exercises, as these help ease the tension in the spine. Throughout the day, the spine holds up your head for several hours, and it can lead to a build-up of stress. It's good to do exercises or asanas that encourage you to hold your head downwards, such as downward dog, to relieve the pressure. It also improves blood flow to the body and acts like a natural facial. You'll probably look a bit flushed afterwards, but it's also extremely beneficial for the skin.

I hope I've given you enough ideas on how to structure what you work into your fitness routine each week and month. Remember to breathe, get the posture correct, consistently work in variations and keep yourself engaged and challenged, so that you can keep working towards your individual goal.

The When of It

My recommendation would be to exercise early in the day, as you have more energy when you wake up. It's best not to work out a tired body. However, this is something I encourage everyone to figure out according to what makes them feel best. Some people love the stress buster that exercise can be after a day of work. If you feel like you enjoy working out in the evening, stick to that. Listen to your body.

Don't work out in the morning if you've woken up feeling sluggish or tired.

The How Much of It

I never tell people how many reps of an exercise to do. I don't even decide it for myself. The basic rule is, do it a little beyond when you start feeling the burn in your muscles. For some people, it might happen at 10 reps, for others at 20 reps. It might differ for the same person even from one day to another, depending on their fitness levels, their goals, how well rested they are, what they ate and how much they exercised the day before.

Also be careful of how often you exercise. If you work out too much, it can have an adverse effect and cause the body to release cortisol, which is a stress hormone, and can lead to weight gain. If you feel like you need to skip a day, that's okay too. By constantly thinking of how you must work out, you might be putting unnecessary pressure on yourself, which the body perceives as stress and releases cortisol.

All these challenges you see on social media that encourage 100 days of working out are good to keep you motivated, but not if you are obsessing over working out every day. Moreover, if you're not resting in between, it can be harmful for the body and, sooner or later, you'll make yourself susceptible to injury.

You won't gain weight or become unhealthy if you don't work out for a couple of days. Go easy on yourself when you need to and don't obsess. Good fitness and being in balance with your body is just as much about enjoying the exercise you do.

How Much Rest Do You Need?

There are two main types of rest, and you need to make sure you get enough of both. Active rest is when you don't do a fixed workout that day but indulge in light activities, such as walks and stretches. Passive rest is complete rest and accounts for the amount of sleep you get. For both kinds of rest, don't forget the mind. If you're constantly worrying about something on your rest day or thinking ahead to what needs to be done the next day, the body will hold on to stress and release cortisol.

Everyone should get between seven to nine hours of sleep every night, so that all the chemical, hormonal and anti-inflammatory responses can be at their peak level. Sleep is critical for those who lift weights and train for any activity, so that protein can build and repair the damaged muscles. Sleep also keeps your immune system functioning at a high level to fight off sickness.

It is better to sleep at the same time every day so that you don't disrupt your routine. Sleep in the most natural setting possible, with as few artificial lights as possible. Wake up with the sun if possible. Here are a few suggestions to maximize the rest you get:

Relax: Activities such as meditation and yoga will relax your body and mind and prepare you for bedtime. A few yoga poses actually help you get better sleep. There are balasana, bhujangasana, eka pada rajakapotasana, setu bandha sarvangasana, supta matsyendrasana and viparita karani.

Turn off gadgets: TVs, computers, laptops, cell phones, video games and tablets emit artificial blue light that can affect your body's production of melatonin and, in turn, your quality and quantity of sleep. It is best to keep them away from you as soon as you hit the bed.

Journal: Your mind should be at rest to give you good sleep. Write down whatever has bothered you throughout the day so you don't think of it after you have turned off the lights.

When you understand your sleep habits better, and the amount of quality sleep you get each night improves, you can begin to alter your habits and enhance your sleep and overall health. If you're having trouble sleeping at night, try drinking camomile tea or apply lavender oil on your temples or your forehead before sleeping. Practising the corpse pose, shavasana, before sleeping helps improve the sleep cycle too. During this asana, your breathing slows down and your blood pressure drops. This is how the mind and body both relax, which results in better sleep.

Specific Goals

Wherever I go, the topic of conversation invariably turns to the latest workout regime or new diet. And they're all centred on weight. Most people are trying to lose weight while a few are trying to gain weight. I feel slightly annoyed with such conversations, as there's so much more to wellness than weight loss, programmes and pills. When you're fit, weight loss follows naturally. When you have your routine in place and you're eating right, your body will lose the extra fat it is holding on to. Similarly, if you train regularly and eat enough protein, you will gain weight the right way.

Most people do their workout and then eat junk or sit on the couch for the rest of the day. And then they complain that they've put on weight. Learn to be active through the day. For example, I work out in the mornings and go for a walk in the evening, which lets me spend some time in nature too. Or every time I get a phone call, I walk up and down the room I'm in or do some stretches.

How to Achieve Your Ideal Weight

I gained cellulite for the first time during the lockdown because I couldn't do any weight training and intense cardio, but I didn't fuss over it as I knew I would lose it with a couple of months of regular training at the gym.

Before you read on, I'd like to stress again that both vital and secondary foods affect the body. Weight is only a small piece of the wellness puzzle. Placing too much emphasis on body weight can cause areas of vital food to suffer. More often than not, I have observed that the obsession with weight creates a stressful relationship with food as well as physical activity.

Rather than getting caught up in the number on the weighing scale, focus on balancing your vital food and making good secondary food choices. The rest will fall in place and it will be easier for you to reach your ideal weight. Keep in mind the following things:

1. **Switch your beverages**

    Weight loss: Add more water to your diet to contribute to weight loss over time, because an increase in water intake may reduce calorie intake. Replace colas and packaged juices with water because those drinks only have empty calories.

Weight gain: If you're looking to add more calories to your diet, smoothies packed with whole foods are a great option. Smoothies can help add calories between meals. Try using nut butters, flaxseeds, chia seeds and avocados.

2. **Eat nutrient-dense food**

Weight loss: A well-rounded diet based on whole foods can naturally help support a healthy weight. Food with healthy fats, complex carbohydrates and lean proteins will give you the adequate nutrition and also make you feel fuller. Fibre from plants keeps you fuller for longer, so you're less likely to reach for snacks after meals. They also benefit gut health, which has an effect on a person's weight.

Weight gain: Eat several small meals that include whole foods instead of going for larger meals. Snacks such as nuts and seeds, dried fruits and cheese help add calories. Include high-quality fat sources, such as olive and coconut oils and salmon during meals.

3. **Manage stress**

Weight loss: Stress causes weight to increase in two ways: The body increases its production of stress hormones, which is why the body starts to store fat. Stress also leads people to often seek comfort in fatty, sugary foods.

Weight gain: While some gain weight due to stress, others notice a decrease in appetite, thus causing weight loss. If you are one of them, make an effort to eat regular meals with others and include interesting spices and flavours in your cooking. Ginger and cayenne are known to stimulate appetite. People who tend to be more hyper struggle to gain weight sometimes because of constant stress. They should do activities like yoga and meditation to calm themselves down. The chapter on spirituality will tell you more on how to go about it.

4. **Prioritize sleep**

   Weight loss: Skipping sleep can cause disruptions in your circadian rhythm, which can increase inflammation in the body and create conditions conducive to weight gain. Sleep deprivation also causes your body to produce more ghrelin, the hormone that signals you to eat.

   Weight gain: Your body rests and repairs itself when you sleep, so it can be more effective during the day. Add calories throughout the day, but try not to eat at least two to three hours before bedtime, as this may affect your sleep quality.

5. **Exercise**

   Weight loss: Working out relieves stress, burns calories and gives your metabolism a boost even when you're not working out. Make sure to have some protein-rich food after your workout to help support muscle repair.

Weight gain: Resistance exercises and strength training can help build muscle. But eat enough calories to support your workout. A protein-rich meal following a workout will also support muscle repair.

Any effort to reach your ideal weight should not include starving yourself. All bodies need a certain amount of protein, nutrients and fats to function. Eating too little will slow down your metabolism and cause the body to retain fat. So starving yourself is counterproductive. Eating less than 1,200 calories a day is extremely unhealthy.

Always remember that your ideal weight is the weight that lets you live happily and in good health. It is a number that works for you—it's not something a beauty magazine, your parents or friends can decide for you. If you are getting most of your calories from real, non-processed food, exercising at least three to five days a week, avoiding prolonged periods of sitting, getting between seven to eight hours of sleep and maintaining strong social and family relationships, I'm sure you are already at your ideal weight. It's best to not obsess over a number and do the best that you can to reach it—whether it is by losing a few kilos or gaining a few.

Building Abs

Getting a six-pack is something that requires a lot of hard work, discipline, dedication and proper nutrition. You'll have to be very careful about the food you eat and consistently work to bring down the body-fat percentage. When you lose flab around the midriff, the muscle definition will begin to show. You'll have to do a lot of core work to strengthen the muscles. Chart out the progress before you begin, so that you know what you have to do and don't get discouraged early on. Make sure your diet includes the right proportion of lean protein, good carbs and healthy fats, and that you cut out junk food.

Losing Inches around the Hips, Thighs and Waist

A lot of women I know have these specific goals in mind when they start working out. While cardio is good to get you started, inch loss won't happen unless you're doing strength training and body-weight exercises. It becomes very important to do enough reps of squats, lunges, leg lifts and planks in this case. Make sure you don't neglect working out the other parts of the body. You can find below some common exercises you can do. I haven't mentioned the reps or how long you should do them, because that depends on your goals and your fitness levels. I suggest you start with a fewer number of reps and increase the reps and the sets as you get fitter and stronger.

To tone your inner thighs:

Curtsy lunges
Lunges with dumb-bells
Pile squats
Medicine ball side lunges

For a slimmer waist:

Jumping oblique twists
Russian twists

Pilates side planks with leg raises
Crisscross crunches
Windshield wipers

To burn hip fat:

Squats
Side lunges
Fire hydrants
Wall sits
Banded walks
Step-ups with weights
Side-lying leg raises

Final Thoughts

Wellness is what you sustain day after day. When you are in balance, you feel strong, motivated, unstoppable, joyous and fit. It'll be a source of vital food and will give you satisfaction like nothing else. Don't just go all out to achieve your goal and lose sight of your health in the process. Physical fitness is more than just having strong arms or a toned stomach. It's about self-care, good health and a positive, strong mind at the end of the day. Learn to rest when you need to and push yourself on the days you're just being lazy. When you get to the point where you're in sync with your body, you'll be in balance. See how it'll help all the other pieces of your life fall into place as well.

How I Stay Fit

Here's the schedule I maintain every week to stay healthy and focused on my physical fitness. This plan works for me. You can give it a try or work out your own modifications to it, as long as all your body parts are feeling the burn. I follow this schedule for a few months and then change it a bit to make sure I continue staying active and injury-free. And even while doing this workout, I add a variety of exercises every week. I change the accessories or machines. I add outdoor training, pool workouts, beach or park workouts, animal movements— the list is endless. My workouts are my playground.

Day 1: Upper body

I use dumb-bells or barbells to work on my back, both upper and lower, shoulders (shoulder presses), chest and arms (mostly body-weight triceps and dips, along with bicep curls—both regular and preacher curls).

Day 2: Yoga

I love yoga; it is one of my favourite forms of exercise. My yoga, too, is different each time. Each sequence is different from the last one. I do what comes to mind at that time without thinking much.

Day 3: Lower body

This is the day to focus on my glutes. I do exercises such as donkey kicks and free weights. I also do deadlifts and front squats, or use some bands.

Day 4: Cardio

This includes any kind of cardio exercise I am in the mood for. It is usually a power walk on the treadmill but I can also opt for the elliptical or rower if I am indoors. If I am outdoors, I cycle or do a one-and-a-half-hour uphill and downhill brisk walk.

Day 5: Rest

My body needs to recover from everything I have challenged it to over the past four days, so Day 5 of the week is for rest.

Day 6: Whole body

I do push-ups and combine these with squats, standing rolls and a shoulder press. I also work on my abs by planking and doing different variations of planks, such as leg kicks or spider planks, as well as leg lifts and side twists.

Day 7: Yoga

I end my week with yoga again because it calms me and relaxes my mind, leaving me looking forward to the coming week.

SPIRITUALITY

Release, allow, flow and grow.

When I returned to Mumbai after my time at the detox centre, I felt rejuvenated. The daily treatments and the food had done wonders for my body, but I was also lucky to have had the most extraordinary experiences that nourished my soul. On one of my morning walks, I encountered a 300-year-old mango tree. Despite the age, it bore fruit. I stood in awe the first time I saw it. I couldn't keep away from it for the rest of my stay. I began having my breakfast while facing the tree and would spend several minutes every day hugging its magnificent trunk. I'd shut my eyes, take deep breaths and feel the vibrations flowing from the tree to my body. At the end of those few minutes, I would feel a divine calm, something I have rarely experienced. Even birds gravitated towards it. The peacocks and peahens, which had hundreds of acres to roam about, would walk towards this tree at sunset, spend the night on it and fly away in the morning. There were many other trees they could spend the night on. But why this tree? It must've been some kind of spiritual connection.

It is one thing to exist with nature and another to understand how we all coexist as part of a larger consciousness. We are so used to the confines of society that we rarely pay attention to the spiritual value of things. We overlook the fine balance of the ecosystem around us and how we all play a part in it. So many species are suffering as a result of our actions, which have led to the destructive complications of climate change. For example, declining bee populations across the world will affect the crucial role they play in pollination, which will have a ripple effect on crop production and weather.

Everything around us has a unique vibration. Trees too. When we hug or touch them, their specific vibrations affect our well-being. I know many people are likely to dismiss my experience as mumbo jumbo. Even I couldn't have imagined the depth of it until I truly felt it. When I hugged that tree, I felt one with nature. I've been at peace in the outdoors from a very young age, but the experience of hugging that tree made me realize that what I felt was a deep, spiritual connection.

Spirituality is a wide-ranging concept. But at its core, it is about connecting to something larger than ourselves. It helps us answer the question that all of us have, at some point, asked, no matter our beliefs and convictions: What is the meaning of the life we have been given?

Some people find that their spiritual life is linked to their religion or a place of worship—a temple, a church, a mosque, a synagogue, or any other place they choose to worship at. Some find succour in a personal relationship with God or a higher power. Others look for meaning in nature or art. Some find it in yoga or meditation. For me, spirituality is in all of these, along with a keen sense of being alive, stress-free and connected to others. I have found that my definition of spirituality has changed as I have matured, thanks to my experiences and relationships.

There are several ways I practise spirituality—
grounding, forest-bathing, prayer, gratitude, yoga,
meditation and so much more. Here are some of the ways
in which you, too, could incorporate spirituality into
your life.

Grounding

We are bioelectrical beings living on an electrical planet.
Our cells transmit multiple frequencies that run our heart,
immune system, muscles and nervous system. Just like
electrical appliances, humans need earthing, or grounding.
When we connect directly with the ground, by walking
barefoot on soil, sand or grass, it helps balance the electrical
charges in our body. I know this sounds incredible, but it's
true. Throughout the day, we are in contact with electrical
appliances or surfaces that cause our body to build up
a positive charge. To strike a balance, we need to stay
connected with the earth. When the human body comes
in contact with the earth, electrons automatically flow
from the body (positively charged) to the earth (negatively
charged) to me.

Grounding isn't a recent wellness trend but an age-old
practice. Here are some of its numerous benefits:

Neutralizes free radicals: Free radicals are generated
through inflammation, infection, cell damage, trauma,
stress and a toxic environment. These cause damage
to our cells and our DNA. Grounding is a simple and
inexpensive way in which most of us can keep these
destructive forces at bay.

Improves our sleep cycle and helps manage stress: Grounding helps establish normal cortisol levels, which results in sound sleep and reduced stress levels.

Improves cardiovascular health: A study published in the *Journal of Alternative and Complementary Medicine* found that grounding can reduce the risk of cardiovascular disease and heart attacks.[1] It also helps maintain healthy blood pressure levels. Holistic experts recommend at least fifteen minutes of grounding every day for patients suffering from high blood pressure.

Helps keep premature ageing at bay: Free radicals are the root cause of premature ageing. It causes our skin to wrinkle and body to weaken. Grounding can help us strike a balance. When we connect with the earth, our body starts to get back to its natural, neutral and balanced state.

Helps raise your energy levels: Practising grounding regularly can make you feel fresh and energetic. Connecting with the earth can also help you connect with your inner self. We also need good bacteria from the earth, which we can get through grounding.

Forest-bathing

Imagine a forest—majestic trees rising towards the bright blue sky, sunrays descending and mingling with the green of

---

[1] Gaétan Chevalier et al, 'Earthing (Grounding) the Human Body Reduces Blood Viscosity—a Major Factor in Cardiovascular Disease', *Journal of Alternative and Complementary Medicine*, 2013, https://www.ncbi.nlm.nih.gov/pmc/articles/PMC3576907/ (accessed on 31 July 2020).

the forest, reflected in the dewdrops on the leaves. You sit on a log of wood with your eyes closed and your mind open as you inhale the fresh air mixed with the scent of the forest. You listen to leaves rustling and birds chirping as you feel the warmth of the sun and the cool, gentle wind brushing against your skin.

This is the essence of forest-bathing. Every time I visit a detox centre, I try to make sure it is located in serene surroundings that I can enjoy. I've noticed that my love for nature is something I have passed on to my kids as well. My son can sit for hours in our lawn among the trees that my father-in-law had grown and taken care of. Maybe it is a way for him to connect with his grandfather and feel the vibrations flow from those trees to him.

Forest therapy was first developed in Japan during the 1980s and has now become an important subject in preventive healthcare and Japanese medicine. The Japanese government spent $4 million promoting forest-bathing programmes between 2004 and 2012.[2] It is called shinrin–yoku in the country and refers to all activities that involve visiting the forest for therapeutic benefits.

Several experiments have been conducted to learn how forest-bathing positively affects the human body. Certain studies have concluded that the scents released by trees, produced from phytoncides, have a great impact on the human body. Phytoncides are natural oils secreted by plants.

---

[2] Ephrat Livni, 'Japanese "Forest Medicine" Is the Science of Using Nature to Heal Yourself—Wherever You Are', Quartz, 21 February 2008, https://qz.com/1208959/japanese-forest-medicine-is-the-art-of-using-nature-to-heal-yourself-wherever-you-are/ (accessed on 17 August 2020).

They are part of its defence mechanism against insects, fungi, algae and bacteria. It is said that phytoncides help with conditions such as depression and anxiety by curbing the production of stress hormones. Certain studies also state that phytoncides boost natural-killer-cell activity and aid the production of anti-cancer proteins in the body.[3]

Walking into the woods engages all our senses—sight, smell, hearing, touch and taste. Taking it all in boosts the immune system, reduces cortisol levels, helps with insomnia, lowers blood pressure, improves respiratory function, slows down the heart rate, reduces symptoms of hyperactivity, decreases risk of cardiovascular diseases, increases energy levels, accelerates recovery and boosts concentration and mindfulness. Phew! That's a lot of benefits. I hope this convinces you to forest-bathe too.

If a forest isn't accessible, you can even drive to a park or a wooded area. Just switch off your mobile phone, ditch all your gadgets for a few hours and take in the atmosphere around you. Sit down, take deep breaths and be in the moment. You could even use it as an opportunity to practise grounding. There's no Wi-Fi in the forest, but you'll surely find a strong connection.

Nature

When day-to-day life takes its toll, I turn to nature. Increasing my spiritual connection with nature is just the

---

[3] Qing Li, 'Effect of Forest Bathing Trips on Human Immune Function', *Environmental Health and Preventive Medicine*, 2010, https://www.ncbi.nlm.nih.gov/pmc/articles/PMC2793341/ (accessed on 31 July 2020).

tonic I need to rejuvenate myself. It reminds me that there is a beautiful world out there. I feel so inconsequential in the face of nature that all my worries and stress drain away. Every time I travel outside the city, I ensure I find a place every night to star-gaze. Lying on the ground or grass and looking up at the night sky makes me calm. I also get excited to relive school geography lessons and try to guess the correct names of the stars and constellations. When I'm in Mumbai, I love going to parks where I can see colourful butterflies and other birds.

My children have grown up around beaches, because every holiday we went to was a beach holiday. We all love spending the day in the water and walking on sand. Swimming in the sea is therapeutic, as it is rich in other mineral salts such as sodium and iodine. While most people either love beaches or mountains, I love them both equally, because both give me the chance to spend time in nature.

Breathing

You may wonder why I have linked breathing to spirituality. Over the years, I've practised deep-breathing and reaped immense benefits from it. It's helped my body, but I also find it one of the best ways to calm my mind and reach a place of spirituality. It particularly helps me manage stress, which can crop up every now and then, and has been a soothing effect in times of distress. The way I see it, life is all about finding ways to handle the problems it throws at us. Connecting with the self and being spiritual is the one fool-proof method that works for everyone.

Some people have a tendency to hold their breath when they are stressed. Others take shallow breaths. As a result, less oxygen enters the body and bloodstream, and an even lesser amount goes to the brain. Stress causes shallow breathing and this, in turn, aggravates stress. Because of this, only the upper part of your lungs are used, less oxygen gets in and more carbon dioxide builds up. This can result in panic attacks, or a feeling of lethargy and sluggishness.

The yogic breathing technique of pranayama helps immensely. Other cultures, too, have their own word to describe the importance of breathing to attain a spiritual life. In Japan it's called *ki*; in China *qi*. Certain tribes in Africa call it *num*. The ancient Hawaiians called it *ha*. In Hebrew, it is referred to as *neshemet ruach chayim*, the spirit of life within the breath. You may be exercising every day and eating healthy food, but if you are breathing wrong, you are more likely to live an unhealthy, stressful life. Follow the steps below a few times a day to breathe fully.

- Hold a hand to your chest and another to your belly, so you can feel both contract and expand.
- Breathe in slowly till the count of three. Count to four as your breathe out. When you inhale, imagine drawing energy from all around you and also from deep within you at the same time. Focus and gather all that energy in your heart with every inhalation.
- Your stomach should expand as you breathe in and retract as you breathe out.
- When you breathe out, make a 'whoosh' sound through your mouth.

Don't Like Deep-Breathing? There Are Other Ways to Relax

- *The 54321 technique:* Say five things you can see, four things you can touch, three things you can hear, two things you can smell and one thing you can taste. This gives you something to focus on. This is also effective when someone is having a panic attack, and helps the mind calm down.

- *Safe-place meditation:* Decide on a place that makes you feel calm and at peace. Visualize it by including all your senses.

- *Hold a cube of ice:* Because ice provides a sensory shock, it gives you something to focus on. Look at the ice as it melts in your hand. By the time it's water, you'll feel much calmer.

- *Pick up objects near you:* Pick up anything near you, such as your keys. Feel them in your hands. Notice the edges and any changes in texture. This is another way to give your mind something else to focus on.

- *Notice the sounds further away:* Pay attention to the sound that seems farthest from you, and then work inwards, to sounds closer to you. Start with a dog barking in the distance and then the sounds right next to you, such as the utensils being used in the kitchen.

- *A loved one's voice:* Imagine the voice of someone you care about telling you that it is all okay. Ask them to record it for you and listen to it when you are feeling anxious.

Pet Therapy

Those of you who follow me on Instagram must have seen my family's adorable puppy, Peach, featuring in some of the videos. Little Peach is the most wonderful puppy you could ever meet. I'm sure every pet owner feels the same way about theirs, but Peach is truly incredible. He sits by my side when I am feeling low and excitedly jumps all over me every time I enter the house. He loves playing with every guest that comes home and is extremely friendly. He has the brightest personality, even though he didn't have the best start in life. He was the runt of the litter and the last one to be adopted. He is also partially blind in one eye. But you wouldn't know that if you met him. He is such a happy bundle of joy that you can't help but feel exultant in his presence. He doesn't seem at all bothered by his birth defect. He's one of the truest examples of living life to the fullest and spreading happiness one paw at a time.

That's what pets bring to our lives. While one study found that people who owned pets lived longer after a heart attack than those who didn't,[4] another showed that petting one's dog reduced blood pressure. Interacting with animals can also increase people's level of the happy hormone oxytocin.[5] Pets can help improve cardiac health and reduce

---

[4] Bruce Y. Lee, 'Dog Ownership Associated with Longer Life, Here Are the Caveats', Forbes, 12 October 2019, https://www.forbes.com/sites/brucelee/2019/10/12/dog-ownership-associated-with-longer-life-here-are-the-caveats/ (accessed on 17 August 2020).

[5] Andrea Beetz et al, 'Psychosocial and Psychophysiological Effects of Human-Animal Interactions: The Possible Role of Oxytocin', Frontiers in Psychology, 2012, https://www.ncbi.nlm.nih.gov/pmc/articles/PMC3408111/ (accessed on 31 July 2020).

stress. Having a dog as a pet has also been shown to reduce sedentary lifestyle habits in their owners.

Thanks to Peach, I've become a more social person. Hardly a day goes by when I'm not stopped by a stranger who wants to pet Peach when I am out walking him. This invariably leads to a short conversation between me and the other person. I love these little chats, and they brighten up my day every time. They make me feel like I have met a like-minded person, even though I technically know nothing about them. These interactions connect us on a human level, making us more empathetic. I strongly suggest you bring home a pet if you can. It will change your life in a way you didn't even know was possible.

Sound Healing

Sound can set a mood. The soundtrack at the gym gets us moving, for example, while the one in a yoga class promotes quiet concentration. Sound also has a powerful effect on how we feel throughout the day. Our bodies take cues from sounds around us and tell us when to get energized and when to slow down. Chanting and mantra recitation have been part of Indian spirituality for thousands of years. And now research shows that listening to percussion instruments such as gongs, Tibetan singing bowls and tuning forks can reduce stress and place you in a meditative state. It is also said to heal problems such as anxiety, chronic pain, sleep disorders and PTSD.[6]

---

[6] Dawn Kuhn, 'The Effects of Active and Passive Participation in Musical Activity on the Immune System as Measured by Salivary Immunoglobulin A (SIgA)', *Journal of Music Therapy*, 2002, https://pubmed.ncbi.nlm.nih.gov/12015810/ (accessed on 31 July 2020).

Chakras

Chakras refer to the spiritual energy centres in our body. There are seven chakras in us, from the crown of the head, through the neck and along the spine. Each of the chakras corresponds to specific organs as well as physical, emotional, psychological and spiritual states of being. These chakras contain healing energy that keeps us healthy and vibrant.

The root chakra represents our security and survival, as well as money. If this chakra is imbalanced, you might have money issues, fear of moving forward in life and even adrenal fatigue. The sacral chakra represents sexuality and creativity. If this is imbalanced, you will struggle in relationships and connecting with yourself and the world around you. The third chakra is about personal power, and if this is not in balance, you will struggle to stand up for yourself, make your voice heard and be seen. The heart chakra represents love. If it's out of sync, you can either be burning yourself out by being a people-pleaser or you may be so closed off to love that you self-sabotage all relationships. The throat chakra represents your voice. When it's not in balance, you'll often feel like you aren't being heard. The sixth chakra represents your psychic sight and helps you feel connected to your life. The crown chakra is the representative of your spiritual connection. It signifies your connection to love yourself.

One of the best ways to balance your chakras and find lasting peace and calm is to chant. Repeating a mantra that you feel close to creates vibrations in your chest, lower abdomen and throat. This sets up a pattern of energy that can nurse your ailing energy fields back to health. Yoga, too, can open blocked chakras by manipulating the various parts of the body associated with the chakra through poses designed to stimulate these energy centres.

Crystals

Everything in the universe has its own unique energy. Even a solid object, such as a chair, absorbs and reflects energy, though it may be in minuscule amounts. It may not look like that to the naked eye, but healing crystals and the cells in our body are made up of the same kind of energy. Just like magnets use energy to attract or repel, healing stones crystals do too. When you place crystals over certain parts of your body, your energy moves in accordance with the properties of the crystal, and can help with everything from headaches to anxiety. Crystals have the ability to absorb and remove certain types of energy from the body. They can also push energy into the body and the mind. One of their best qualities is their ability to bring about balance. Sometimes, your energy may be misaligned, and healing crystals are used to balance out disharmony in energies. You can even put a crystal in a bottle and add drinking water to it—the water will be full of good energy. Knowing which crystal is right for you depends on your energies. To learn more about it, seek an expert's opinion.

Prayer

Every night for the past few years now I perform a ritual before I get into bed. Along with praying for the good health and well-being of my family and friends, I say a few lines in my mind. I learnt them at school and they have somehow stuck. It goes like this:

> *Every morning when the day has begun, I thank God*
>   *for all He has done*
> *Every evening I kneel to pray, thank you God for*
>   *another day*
> *Thank you for the sun, my God, thank you for the*
>   *moon*
> *Thank you for the days and nights, mornings and*
>   *afternoons*
> *Thank you for my companions, God, who cheer me*
>   *when I'm down*
> *Thank you for the people, God, wherever they are found.*

These words calm me down and help bring order to my thoughts. I may not be a regular at church, but God is never far from me. I believe that God is within all of us and we carry Him with us wherever we go. He is in the smile of children, in the beauty of nature and within the hearts of the people we love. Prayer helps me connect deeper to my spiritual self because it is a time of reflection, reassurance and rejuvenation. I think of it as a spiritual reset button. It reminds me of all the beautiful things we have to be grateful for.

Gratitude

The prayer I say every night isn't to ask for things—it is to express gratitude for all I am and all I have. It's about letting the universe know that I have a wonderful life and a time for counting my blessings and good fortune. There are so many benefits of gratitude that I believe it deserves a book of its own, but I'll focus on a few.

Studies have found that if you are grateful, you are less resentful towards someone who has something you don't.[7] It helps you recover more quickly from stress and adversity by helping you interpret negative events. Thinking about the things I have rather than focusing on what I don't always gives me perspective and leaves me feeling better about my life and circumstances.

All of us can write a long list of how life has wronged us, can't we? But how about we make a list of all the wonderful things and people we already have in our lives? It could be the love of your parents, friends who cheer you every step of the way, a career that satisfies you, a safe and comfortable place to live in or just a nice experience that's made you a better person. I am so grateful that I get to work in a field I am passionate about—physical and mental fitness. My family and friends are healthy, and my two children have grown up to be lovely and kind human beings. When we take a moment to pause and count our blessings, even in a difficult moment, we realize that our cup always runs over.

Another benefit of gratitude is that it makes you more helpful, empathetic, spiritual, religious, forgiving and less materialistic. Gratitude also increases your sense of self-worth immensely and helps you avoid the negative trap of constantly blaming yourself and comparing yourself to others. Keep a gratitude journal—I'm sure you'll feel happier and less anxious, and it'll help you sleep better.

Also, every time you feel particularly grateful towards someone, try to write them a thank-you letter and mention

---

[7] Robert Emmons, 'Why Gratitude Is Good', Greater Good Magazine, 2010, https://greatergood.berkeley.edu/article/item/why_gratitude_is_good (accessed on 31 July 2020).

the reasons for it. They will receive a happy surprise when they read the letter, and you will feel so wonderful for having shared your feelings.

On days when ten things go bad, I make it a point to feel grateful for the one or two things that have gone right. I believe that even on a crappy day, a bright spot can be found. Why sit in a dark room, when all you need to learn is how to switch on the light? All that is required is that you are able to identify when something good happens to you. For me, it could be something as simple as my dog sitting on my lap or my husband cooking for me. These are usually life's most overlooked, yet important blessings.

Charity and Giving Back

Bill Gates has pledged to donate most of his $110-billion fortune to charity because he wants to contribute to the world. Explaining his decision to not leave any of it to his two children, Gates said, 'It's like saying which children are most important.'[8] Investor Warren Buffet, too, has pledged to give away most of his wealth. In fact, Gates and Buffet have together managed to get forty of the world's wealthiest entrepreneurs—including Oracle founder Larry Ellison and *Star Wars* creator George Lucas—to sign up for the Giving Pledge charity initiative, whereby billionaires agree to donate huge chunks of their fortunes to charity.

---

[8]   Sophie Borland, 'Bill Gates Pledges to Leave His £30 Billion Fortune to Charity . . . Rather Than His Children', *Daily Mail*, 20 June 2008, https://www.dailymail.co.uk/news/article-1027878/Bill-Gates-pledges-58-billion-fortune-charity--children.html (accessed on 31 July 2020).

According to a study by the University of Oregon, people donate to charity because it leaves them feeling good.[9] The study used brain-imaging technology on volunteers as they donated money to a food bank. Results showed that the pleasure centres of the brain were activated by the process of giving. Researchers contend that the study supports the idea of a feeling similar to a 'warm glow' and that people are willing to act in the service of others, even if it does not directly benefit them.

One of the major positive effects of donating time, money or belongings is simply feeling good about giving. Being able to give to those in need helps you achieve a greater sense of personal satisfaction and growth. Studies show that charity has a positive impact on the brain. These effects are similar to activities people usually associate with joy and happiness, such as eating and exercising, or affectionate gestures such as giving someone a hug.

According to me, the impact is unexplainable. Just knowing that you can help someone reach somewhere, or help someone be something, is incredibly satisfying in a way almost nothing else is. Giving back to society is uplifting. Giving need not only be monetary—it can be through your time and actions too. It can even be in speaking up, voicing your opinions and making more people aware.

You can always give nutritious food or clean clothes to the poor man begging at your car window instead of turning him away with the justification that 'they don't actually get

9   William T. Harbaugh, Ulrich Mayr and Daniel R. Burghart, 'Neural Responses to Taxation and Voluntary Giving Reveal Motives for Charitable Donations', *Science*, 2007, https://pubmed.ncbi.nlm.nih.gov/17569866/ (accessed on 31 July 2020).

any of the money, it's all part of a larger game—they're scamming you'.

It's easy to turn a blind eye to other people's problems, but if you can just take some time out and get involved in helping those who need it, it would set in motion a trail of kindness that may find its way back to you someday.

I give back by helping people better their health. My social media pages are full of motivation, whether it is signature workouts or health tips and positivity. A number of people get in touch with me after looking at my social media posts, telling me how the information I have put up has helped them get healthier and stronger. The feeling I get when I hear positive feedback is indescribable.

Yoga

Finally, we come to my favourite form of spirituality. What can I say about yoga that the world doesn't already know? When I started practising yoga and meditation twenty-five years ago, people used to look at me incredulously. They would make fun of me and loudly wonder how such a slow form of exercise could compete with the sweat-drenched workouts at the gym.

Well, we all know the benefits of yoga now, don't we? I think it should be made compulsory in all schools. It's not easy being a kid in school these days. They witness a lot more violence and bullying—and pressure to succeed, at all costs. If they have access to yoga from a young age, they will have the tools they need to handle the challenges that being an adult brings.

Thanks to yoga, I am fitter, calmer and less stressed— and the energy to rival people half my age. I also don't get triggered easily by things that used to upset me very easily. I cannot imagine life without yoga any more.

Yoga involves concentration on the breath and the body, which makes it a great way to soothe the mind and relieve it of worries. It has been proven to reduce anxiety and depression. According to a Harvard University article, yoga helps regulate a person's stress-response system. With its ability to lower blood pressure and heart rate, as well as improve respiration, yoga provides us with the means to deal with anxiety and depression. Multiple studies have shown that yoga can decrease the secretion of cortisol, the stress hormone, and reduce inflammation. Like spirituality, yoga is a personal activity, yet universally beneficial. Many start practising it to have a toned body but stay with it as it becomes an anchor on their path of life. Its effects go deeper and speak to the spiritual side of you.

Last year, for about three months, my workout consisted of strength training, endurance and calisthenics. I wanted to see how far I could push my body. In the process, yoga took a back seat. I didn't practise it as much as I usually would. But soon enough, my body and mind began telling me that it was time to go back to my first love. While the endurance training at the gym was making my body stronger, the calming effect that yoga brought was absent. I could feel myself getting irritated at minor issues. It showed me that we needed to continually practise yoga for it to bring us its benefits. I have now vowed to never put it on the back burner. I use it as daily medicine.

Meditation

Mindfulness means using your senses to focus on the exact moment you are in and making the most of it. The best way I have found to be mindful is by practising meditation. It's easy because anyone can learn to meditate with a few simple guidelines. However, it is also extremely difficult, because in our increasingly hectic and stressful world—where smartphones, social media and constant connectivity lead to burnout, insomnia and loneliness—it is a concept we have to work on every day to master. I have been meditating for more than twenty-five years now—that one practice of shutting down the thoughts that clutter the mind and can ruin one's well-earned balance. It has seen me through a lot in life—the everyday realities of marriage, the joys and frustrations of raising kids in an unkind world, career growth and setbacks, and the loss of people I held close to my heart. I have been able to cope with all of this because my mind always functions like a well-oiled machine. There is no fog, no hesitation, no deliberation and definitely no stress that interferes with what needs to be done. That is the power of meditation. I'm going to help you get started right away. Once you are comfortable with it, you can increase the amount of time you spend each day on meditation.

- Get into a comfortable position. It could be on a chair or cross-legged on the floor.
- Close your eyes and take a deep breath.
- Clear your mind. This is a lot harder than it seems and will take a lot of practice. But it will happen if you persist. You will start out strong. Your mind will be empty for a second before a stray thought enters. You let it appear and then push it out.
- After a while, another thought will appear. You let it unravel and then push it out. Thoughts will keep jumping in and out of your mind.

- That is why try meditating first for just five minutes. Then increase it to ten minutes and more as you feel yourself getting better at it.
- You are unlikely to succeed the first few times you try it. But it will get easier. Just keep pushing thoughts out as soon as they try to enter your mind.

There are other ways to meditate too.

1. *Mindfulness meditation:* Here, you pay attention to your thoughts. You don't become involved with them; you just observe and take note of patterns.
2. *Spiritual meditation:* Spiritual meditation is similar to prayer. You reflect on the silence around you and seek a deeper connection with God.
3. *Focused meditation:* It involves concentration using any of the five senses—touch, sight, hearing, smell and taste.
4. *Movement meditation:* Movement meditation includes walking through the woods, gardening and other gentle forms of motion.
5. *Mantra meditation:* This uses a repetitive sound to clear the mind. It can be a word, a phrase or a sound, such as 'Om'.
6. *Transcendental meditation:* This one is the most popular type of meditation. Here, a mantra or a series of words is used, which can be specific to the individual.

Walking Meditation

The COVID-19 virus pushed us all indoors. And while so many people exercised at home, they probably weren't as mindful of their mental health as well. Pacing is a wellness practice and by slowing it down, it can becomes a destressing activity. While meditating in a sitting position, we focus on our breathing, whereas in walking meditation, the focus is on the movement of our body. Here are the six steps of walking meditation.

- Before you begin, feel the sensation of your feet on the ground. Take a deep breath and, as you exhale, begin to walk.
- Start by walking at a normal pace. Slowly bring the mind into the body and notice how the body feels as you walk.
- Notice the movement of your body, including the arms, legs, hands and feet. Observe the movement of your legs.
- Gradually, slow your pace down a little. Pay attention to the sensation of your soles pressing against the floor. Feel one foot pressing down, then the pressure easing off as you lift the foot. Then feel the next foot pushing down.
- Be aware of the space around you. Walk slower as you continue to concentrate on the sensation of one foot and then the other.
- Continue for as long as you want, and when you finish, stop and take a big, deep breath.

Final Thoughts

I remember a scene from one of my favourite movies, *Zindagi Na Milegi Dobara*. In it, the three friends go deep-sea diving in Spain, with Hrithik Roshan's character, who is scared of water, going underwater for the first time in his life. I saw myself in that scene, because I, too, am petrified of water. But over time, I decided to get over my fear, and can now happily say that I have gone scuba diving several times. I still remember the first time I went for it. The silence around stunned me. I knew what to expect, but I still couldn't believe how deafening the silence was. Taking deep breaths, being so aware of each one of them, I took in the magnificent beauty of the ocean. I found it to be the perfect combination of so many activities that help me tap into my spiritual side—being in nature, sound therapy through deep silence, and achieving a mindful and meditative state under water. It helped me connect to the sea like never before. The water was teeming with life, and I had the chance to observe all that beauty as a quiet spectator. Even the smallest coral was part of a vast system.

I'm pretty sure my expression resembled that of Hrithik's after the dive. He looked shell-shocked—in a good way—as if he couldn't quite believe what he had seen and experienced. Since that first experience, I try to go scuba diving every opportunity I get. I cannot emphasize enough the positive effects of practices that help you tap into your spiritual side, particularly yoga and meditation. Not only do they help you look beyond yourself and gain a deeper understanding of life, but they also take away your stress. And remember, stress-related health problems are responsible for up to 80 per cent of visits to the doctor and account for the third-highest healthcare expenditures, behind only heart disease and cancer.

It might sound ironic that someone whose entire career is built on wellness needs a break from work for precisely that, but that's the truth of it. Every time my body and mind tell me that I need a break, I head to nature. Spending time with the elements and doing these activities that bring me closer to my spiritual self give me a much-needed boost.

I hope I have been able to convey to you how spirituality can help bring about balance in your circle of life. In all my years of seeking mindfulness, I have found that my spiritual side makes me calmer and happier, and feeds my soul. Here are some more tips for you to practise spirituality:

- Sleep, rest and relax. When you're sleep-deprived or stressed, your body craves sugary snacks and caffeine for quick artificial energy.
- Schedule fun time. Boredom and stress can lead to overeating. Make sure to take time to laugh, play and participate in activities you love.
- Take a hot bath. This is a great way to engage the relaxation response and wipe out cortisol, the hormone at the root of weight gain.
- Make your food look beautiful. Use gorgeous dishware and plate your food in a way that's aesthetic. By making meals an event, they will nourish you and fill you up more—both literally and figuratively.
- Hold a baby. Spending time with kids reminds you of the simple wonders of life, and helps you relax and gain perspective.

- Spend time in nature. It connects you with the earth and can provide a natural high. Nature is great at bringing you back to the present moment and can be a source of stress reduction.
- Hug. Humans require physical contact, and long hugs are a great way to get it. They relax you and lead you to produce happy hormones.
- Remember that being calm about everything allows your mind to find solutions. Calm is also a state of trust. Instead of overthinking and overreacting, just surrender for that moment and allow yourself to receive guidance for what doesn't make sense.
- And, finally, spirituality doesn't come from religion. It comes from your soul. Religion is a set of rules, regulations and rituals created by humans, which were supposed to help people spiritually. Due to human imperfection, religion has become corrupt, political, divisive and a tool for gaining power. Spirituality is not theology or ideology. It is simply a way of life—pure and original.

Spirituality is not just about owning crystals or following a trend that may be working for others. It's about connecting with your higher self in a way that expands your consciousness and you can reach your highest potential. The most important thing is to take time out to practise these things. Only then will you be able to tap into your spiritual centre. You are the best person to understand what will work for you and what will help you achieve a sense of balance.

For a Final Dose of Calm, Light a Lamp

If you can, get your hands on the Himalayan pink lamp. These lamps are made of food-grade pure Himalayan salt with a small bulb inside. They purify the air through the process of hygroscopy. They attract water molecules from the environment and absorb them, along with foreign particles such as dust, smoke and pollen, into the salt crystals, leaving the air purified and fresh. They also emit negative ions into the air, which leaves us feeling energetic and enthusiastic. All of this can improve sleep quality.

JOY

Enjoy the little things.

I always think of Bill Gates when I hear of someone struggling to find happiness in life. Gates has probably found the easiest way to that all-elusive goal—giving. As the co-founder of The Giving Pledge, Bill Gates and his wife Melinda have decided to give away 99 per cent of their wealth to those in need. They have called their charitable endeavours the most meaningful work they have done. The act of giving has become a source of true joy in their lives.

Joy is a feeling of great pleasure and happiness. It's a feeling that intensifies when we give. Giving makes us feel happy and induces gratitude. A Harvard Business School report concluded that giving money to someone else makes people happier than spending it on themselves.[1] When people donate money or give someone their time, it activates the parts of the brain associated with pleasure, social

---

[1]   Elizabeth W. Dunn, Lara B. Aknin and Michael I. Norton, 'Prosocial Spending and Happiness: Using Money to Benefit Others Pays Off', Harvard Business School, 2014, https://dash.harvard. edu/bitstream/handle/1/11189976/dunn,%20aknin,%20norton_ prosocial_cdips.pdf?sequence=1 (accessed on 31 July 2020).

connection and trust, and creates a 'warm glow'. Altruism also releases endorphins in the body.

To get the maximum satisfaction from helping others, you need to first figure out what causes you feel most strongly about. It could be helping at your local temple, mosque or church, aiding your house help and their children, civic causes, education or empowerment through sports—basically anything that gives you a few moments of worry before you realize you can actually do something to make it better. My husband is passionate about educating those who don't have easy access to it. With a few supporters, he started a non-profit school in Mumbai. For Mumbai lawyer Afroz Shah, it was the safety of marine animals and the cleanliness of our oceans that mattered. When piles of garbage kept accumulating at a beach near his house, he started cleaning it with his bare hands—and before he knew it, he had thousands of volunteers to help him every weekend. I try to do what I can by educating people about fitness and building a body that can sustain them for many years.

For me, this feeling of absolute joy is almost a constant. My journey to seeking balance through physical fitness, yoga, meditation and spirituality has done wonders for my state of mind and helped me find happiness. That is because my joy is based on how I feel on the inside. Exercising, helping someone do yoga, watching the sun rise, having a healthy family, witnessing my children value life and human connections, and respect the elderly, and seeing them grow up to be empathetic human beings—these are some of the things that make me happy. I don't need material things, such as buying bags or shoes, to make me feel good about myself and my life. In fact, even my son and husband, like me, don't need a lot. My husband is happy with just two pairs of clothes, and my son has followed in his father's footsteps. Ahaan values connections with family and friends more than material things. It brings him joy to give time to his friends and help them when they need it. Hard work, learning a new skill, and even painting and cooking are all sources of joy for my son.

By observing people around me, I have realized that joy can't be found if you are not in touch with your values. People often look at man-made concepts, such as holidays, shopping and gossip, to make themselves happy. They try to fill a void by focusing on the external and not on how they really feel. They don't spend time aligning with their core values. As a result, they manage to temporarily change how they feel, but never truly understand what's causing the feelings in the first place.

I rarely attend parties unless a celebration is involved. But when I do, I always look forward to dancing. All I require at a party to have fun is a dance floor and good music. While others are busy adjusting their designer dresses and fixing their make-up, I am on the dance floor in my jeans, doing mismatched steps. While these same people are checking out the size of the diamonds others are wearing, I am looking for people with big smiles to connect with. I am carefree, because I have figured out what really matters to me. I have always felt responsible for my own health and happiness, and have invested time in things that make me happy.

I've realized the most important thing is to hold on to your values. What you find to be true, what you know is fair and what you believe in are your values. The more you respect them, the better you will feel about yourself and those you love. Don't be a certain way because society demands it. It's not always necessary to follow the norm, but it's always necessary to follow your heart. Why is it that when we look at children, we feel they are full of innocence? It's because they aren't bound by society's expectations. As we grow older, we look around us and try to adapt in a way that we'd deem fit for the people around us. But in doing that, we lose our innocence and ourselves in the process. To truly be yourself, you need to let go of preconceived notions and do what resonates with you.

Finding and Spreading Joy

My husband often tells us a story about tying a thread to a dragonfly and watching it fly when he was a child. He's told us this tale a number of times—an indication of how much fun he had while doing it—and we enjoy hearing about it every time. We all did such innocent things in our childhood, a time when we had no stress or worries, and all we thought about was playing with our friends after coming back from school. It was a time of unadulterated joy in our lives, which we lost as we grew older, as life found ways to pull us down. It was a time we trusted people without asking them to prove themselves and immersed ourselves in these little wonders. But over time, we have slowly become desensitized to the things that once brought us joy.

I want us all to regain that sense of wonder, to be awed by the little things in our grown-up lives. Just because birds chirp every day does not make it any less beautiful. By regaining your intrigue and wonder for all the little things in life, you will slowly realize what brings you joy. It's always the simple things that pack the biggest feelings. Doing this every moment, every day, will make you truly happy. You will know yourself better, and this may even help you choose a career of your choice or figure out who you truly enjoy spending time with. You will put yourself at the centre of your life and practise self-love, which has the potential to change your life in the way you want.

So I want you to sit with a piece of paper and a pen, and write down five things that bring you pure, unadulterated joy. Once you've written those down, think deeply about each of them. How can you change your schedule to find time for at least two of these activities on a regular basis? Or is there a way to split your time among these five things? These could be activities that involve doing something for others or just for yourself too.

I have written about the need for self-care in all aspects of life, and I'd like to remind you that without taking care of yourself, it is unlikely that you will find joy. When you make yourself and your needs a priority, you organize your life so that it gives you endless joy. When you use self-care to create a life that you don't want to escape from, you can become more present in the moment. In turn, you come to appreciate every minute in your life, and be happy and grateful for everything you have.

That is the person I have been for a while now. Doing the work I love, surrounding myself with people who uplift me, appreciating the things that really matter, instead of hankering after materialistic stuff—all this has made me the person I always wanted to be. And, in some ways, this has made me a person I never knew I could become. It's been a wonderful journey of a deeper self-awareness. What makes it all the more enlightening and exciting is discovering how it will keep changing my life and the way I react to different situations. Self-love is a big part of my happiness. When you look after yourself, you become a happy person. My life is proof of that.

In moments of immense happiness, does it occur to me that I'm being selfish, especially when there is sadness and misery around me? It doesn't, because I do the most in my power to spread the joy I feel. Contemplating others' sorrow only makes the world a more sorrowful place. I would rather be the reason behind someone's smile. If you are joyous, you can use your joy to lift others out of sorrow, rather than becoming full of sadness yourself.

We live in a culture that demands that we put the happiness of others before ours. But how can an unhappy person make others happy? The concept of self-care is the opposite of selfishness. We need to take care of ourselves first before being capable of caring for others. Once you have found ways to put yourself first, you are naturally more able to extend care to others. This applies in our professional roles and also when we care for friends, family and people in our communities.

Our happiness is affected by those in our social circle. Your joy can influence not one but many around you. Also, we can give ourselves a chance to be happier simply by spending time with happy people. The day I realized this I stopped feeling bad about being happy.

Being joyful does not mean forcing yourself to be happy all the time. The concept of fake-it-till-you-make-it definitely doesn't work here. Instead, you have to actively work towards it to reach a state of bliss. Getting good sleep, exercising and eating right make me feel great. Decluttering does that too, because it clears actual things in front of me and, in turn, clears the cobwebs of my mind.

The benefits of having joy in your life are manifold. I've seen it myself. I started becoming more creative— I painted better than ever before and even designed our entire house with our architect. I also designed the logo and the website of my brand, Balance with Deanne. Joy has also let me control my emotions rather than let my emotions control me. I started developing intimate, deeper relationships with the people in my life, while also believing that these bonds were doing their part in bringing me happiness. I also learnt a lot about myself in the process, which helped me live life on my own terms. And when that started happening, it began to attract all the good things I wanted.

This feeling of joy has impacted every part of my life. In my personal or professional life, I don't judge people— neither do I feel wronged by them. And in one of those rare occasions that I do feel that I have been wronged, I hurt for a while. But over time, I forgive them, because not doing so is a burden on my chest. Forgiving the person and letting them go releases the pain. They may have behaved badly with you because they are themselves unhappy, frustrated or angry with something that's not right in their lives. This open-minded attitude means I see the beauty and goodness in everyone and everything I encounter. If someone looks up at the night sky and sees the cable wires that dot our urban landscape, I see the stars. If someone points out a friend's bad habits, I make sure to list the person's good ones. This persistent desire to find the good in the seemingly bad, and the excitement in the mundane, has led to some people around me labelling me 'too sweet'. People love to believe that a sweet and kind person is too good to be true, and they tend to think the worst—which is, 'This person is just pretending to be this nice', or 'They're fake'. What they don't realize is that goodness and kindness aren't fake when you are happy, secure and content. It won't matter what people say, because your happiness won't be defined in the way theirs is.

Happiness and contentment have also made me hungry for more, but in a positive way. I yearn to learn and grow in my professional life, which has seen my career grow exponentially. I am now more persistent about going after what I want and not wasting my time doing work that doesn't fit in with my purpose. That's how I have the career I do.

It is also joy that has made me brave physically and emotionally. I never learnt to swim—something I wish I had. I have been scared of water ever since my parents took my siblings and me to Juhu beach as children. I remember sitting on a float in just foot-deep water with my sister when a wave crashed into us and toppled us over. I went under for probably a couple of seconds, but I managed to gulp down a lot of water. When I surfaced, I started coughing and was scared I was going to die. That experience put me off swimming completely and I have been scared of water ever since. But once I found balance in my life, I found the courage to go scuba diving and thoroughly enjoyed it. To comfortably swim underwater without any fear was a huge deal for me, especially since I don't even know how to float. But my curiosity and inclination for joy weren't going to let a small thing like fear of water stop me.

It also helps to remember that fear is man-made. Imagine how limitless our actions would be if we didn't allow fear into our lives. Fear stops us from doing things that bring us joy. So be fearless but be mindful and wise about your choices.

I don't have emotional guards in place, because I know that to be truly joyful you have to surrender yourself to the love around you. I love the people in my life fiercely and let them know about it. My heart is always open to them even if I have to risk being hurt sometimes. I have a lot of love to give, but I don't expect it in return. If I don't get the same kind of love from the other person, that's all right. I strongly believe that when you feel love, you become love, and that when joy is a habit, love is a reflex. And that's the only way I know how to live. I learnt this early on, because of the kind of family I grew up in. My father was the only earning member, and we led a very simple life. I have five siblings, and we were all brought up with a focus on the little joys of life, rather than the material things we accumulated through the journey of life. And it is this quality that has taught me to be honest and authentic in every way. I know that joy comes to us because we seek it, despite the grief and heartbreak of the past. I have lost a lot of my family members, including my beloved grandmother, who passed away in front of me when I was quite young. But I strived to remain strong for myself and the others in my family. The loss of my loved ones has only made me more grateful to have had them in my life, and also made me cherish my loved ones and understand their importance in my life.

The link between gratitude and joy is strong. All of us have a lot to be thankful and grateful for in our lives. I am always grateful for my career, which is good for my health and financial freedom. I am thankful that my family and friends are physically healthy and that they choose to love and support me every day.

I encourage you to make your own list of things you believe you are fortunate to have in your life. Just making that list will give you so much joy, because you will be reminded of how wonderful your life is. When we focus on gratitude, a strong current expels the tides of disappointment and releases the tides of love and joy. When we focus on the good and the things we do have, we are more open to receiving joy. To nurture a joyful life is to practise gratitude. It is harder than it sounds because we can't just say, 'I'm going to be more grateful.' It has to be more than just a change in attitude. You have to act on it every day by thinking of the positives when you encounter the ugliness of life.

The best way to seek joy is to find it in the everyday. Know and acknowledge that you have plenty to be thankful for and see the beauty around you. Joy will follow.

HOME-COOKED FOOD

Eat good, feel good.

We've talked about joy and how it forms an important part of the circle of life. Joy comes in all sorts of packages. One of the ways in which I find joy every single day is through the home-cooked food I eat. It looks something like this: I sit on the sofa, hungry and looking forward to eating. My cook walks towards me, with a bowl in his hand—it's food cooked by my husband, the best chef in our house. I look up from my book and my eyes widen in anticipation. As it gets closer, my eyes become bigger, along with my smile. The first bite is soon taken, and I smile my biggest possible smile, appreciating the fresh, flavourful food cooked with love by my husband. I mindfully relish and finish my meal, happy and sated.

There are few things that match the goodness of a plate of healthy, nutritious, home-cooked food. When you shop for the ingredients yourself, picking the best ones, and cook it using your own healthy methods or supervise someone else cooking for you, you know it will be a wholesome meal. Research has shown that people who eat home-cooked meals on a regular basis tend to be happier and healthier, and consume less sugar and processed foods.[1] In the Panday household, my husband, Chikki, doesn't follow any recipes, but instinctively puts together a yummy, healthy—and sometimes unhealthy—dish. He often steps into the kitchen, because our current cook, Subhash, isn't the most talented chef by a mile. Subhash has been with us for many years and when our previous cook—who was better than some Michelin-star chefs—left, he took over the post. We soon realized that cooking is possibly Subhash's weakest skill—he once served us chicken biryani without the chicken because he forgot to add it! But thanks to his goof-ups, we have had quite a few laughs over the years, and also sampled so much more of my husband's cooking. But no matter what, Subhash is part of our family, so despite his lack of cooking talent, he will stay with us as long as he wants to.

The Poison of Processed

I can safely say that more than half the food most of you eat every day is unhealthy, given the quality of ingredients and our food choices. Processed food is the scourge of this generation. Technically, it isn't even food—it is a food-like substance. Despite its easy access and lip-smacking taste, it is incredibly harmful for us.

---

[1] Julia A. Wolfson and Sara N. Bleich, 'Is Cooking at Home Associated with Better Diet Quality or Weight-Loss Intention?', *Public Health Nutrition*, 2015, https://www.cambridge.org/core/journals/public-health-nutrition/article/is-cooking-at-home-associated-with-better-diet-quality-or-weightloss-intention/B2C8C168FFA377DD2880A217DB6AF26F (accessed on 2 August 2020).

Processed food is defined as any food item that has had a series of mechanical or chemical operations performed on it to change or preserve it. It typically comes in a box or a bag, and has a long list of ingredients. To find out if what you're eating is processed, here's a simple test: Look at the ingredients list and ask yourself if it's something you can make at home. If it can only be made in a laboratory or through a chemical process—because it contains ingredients such as high-fructose corn syrup, hydrogenated oil or soya protein isolate—it is highly processed.

Sure, some processed foods can actually be quite healthy, such as precooked whole grains, Greek yoghurt, nut butters and frozen vegetables. Others, however, contain high levels of salt, sugar and fat. Surprisingly, some of the most highly processed foods are advertised as being the healthiest, including low-fat foods, breakfast cereals, whole-wheat bread, frozen meals and condiments. Low-fat foods such as crackers, cookies and salad dressings often have added sugar and salt to make up for flavour, and stabilizers to make up for texture. Some even have more calories than their higher-fat counterparts.

It bodes well to remember that food from a packet will most likely only get stale but not rot. I saw a fascinating video some time ago that showed burgers from seven American fast-food restaurants that had been stored in glass jars for thirty days. In the end, some of them were covered in mould, while others did not look much different from Day 1. Several people have conducted similar experiments where they have stored fast food for a long time, only to realize it just wouldn't go bad. This just shows that processed foods are unnatural and shouldn't be consumed in large quantities. Food is meant to rot naturally. When it doesn't, it has chemicals in it to make it stay that way. And you're consuming them, along with the food, every time.

By cooking at home from scratch, you can cut out all the rubbish that comes with processed food. Its makers are genius marketers and have the world hooked. But we need to remember that the 100 calories you get from a packet of biscuits is not the same as 100 calories from a box of blueberries. Similarly, 200 calories from an aerated drink is nowhere close to the healthy 200 calories you will get from an avocado. My mantra is: If you can't pluck it, peel it or grow it, it isn't good for you.

Know Your Farmer

In India, people know more about Bollywood than the things they put in their and their kids' bodies. It is a sad reflection of our times. It is only when you know what you're eating that you can begin the journey to find balance in your life. Begin by asking your vegetable and fruit vendor where your food is coming from. Once you know, find out how the food is grown and what kind of fertilizers and pesticides are used. Although pesticides are intended to harm only the target pest, if not used correctly, they can harm us too. If there is pesticide residue in your food, it can lead to adverse health problems, including cancer and effects on the reproductive, immune and nervous systems.

Similarly, if you regularly cook meat at home, find out where it is coming from. If it is factory-farmed, it is not healthy. Ideally, the animals should be fed on grass. Try to opt for free-range eggs and meat from animals that are free and not confined to small spaces. Factory-farmed animals are given antibiotics and growth hormones. These wreak havoc on your body when you consume the meat. That is why you should know your farmer and also your food.

Whenever you have the chance and the means, you should opt for organic food. It is healthier, tastier and grown with methods that are kinder to the environment. Organic food should have no added antibiotics, hormones or synthetic additives. Non-organic plants, meanwhile, have higher levels of cadmium, a toxic metal. They also have around four times more pesticide residue than organic food.

Eating food that has been grown without pesticides and chemicals is so rich in nutrients that it will change everything. It can move you from disease to health, from ageing to youth, from death to life.

A common concern while buying organic food is that people don't always know if it really is organic. Look out for the Jaivik Bharat logo and the FSSAI organic logo, as they are allowed to be printed on a product only if it meets certain criteria. However, I don't want you to believe that if you aren't having organic food, you should be ashamed. It is often only available in cities or areas where old methods of farming are being followed. Moreover, it is often more expensive, and not everyone can afford to have it even if they choose to. In such a scenario, I'd recommend washing your food well and adding as many fruits and vegetables to your diet as possible so you make sure you're consuming a whole lot of nutrients.

Switching to unpolished grains and unrefined salt, too, can make a huge difference to your diet. Unpolished grains retain the nutrients that are lost in the polished versions. For example, brown rice contains a whole lot more fibre than polished white rice. Similarly, unrefined salt is a whole food product that is utilized easily by our bodies. It provides minerals, along with important trace minerals that help improve the immune, glandular and nervous systems. I would also suggest using masalas freshly ground with a pestle instead of packet masalas. They are richer in taste and have a shorter shelf life, which is better for your health. We do the same at home. I am quarter east Indian, and growing up, we always had various types of freshly ground bottle masalas at home. The taste is exponentially better than the ready-made packaged masalas available these days. I have held on to this tradition of my community and have taught my cook at home how to make those oh-so-special masalas. Switching to only home-ground masalas also helped me reduce the chronic acidity I was facing.

I'd also like to talk a bit about the kind of oil you use at home for your cooking needs, whether it is for frying, baking, sautéing or drizzling. The first thing to note is its smoke point. An oil's smoke point is when it starts burning and smoking. If you heat oil past its smoke point, it not only affects the flavour, but also reduces the oil's nutritional content. The oil will release harmful compounds called free radicals.

Most oils are nut- or seed-based. As the names suggest, nut oils are extracted from nuts such as almond and groundnut, while seed oils come from seeds of plants such as sunflower and mustard.

Here are some oils that we use on a regular basis in India, and their qualities:

Canola oil: It is derived from rapeseed, a flowering plant, and is pretty healthy and the best for frying, roasting and baking. It is also low in saturated fats.

Extra-virgin olive oil: It is high in heart-healthy monounsaturated fats and best for sautéing and drizzling.

Sunflower oil: This oil is good for deep-frying. It is high in polyunsaturated fats, which have been shown to lower cholesterol, particularly 'bad' LDL cholesterol.

Sesame oil: It is equally high in monounsaturated and polyunsaturated fats, which makes it pretty healthy. It is high in vitamin K, which is great for blood coagulation and bone strength. You can use it as salad dressing or to stir-fry.

Almond oil: This oil is primarily used in baking and making candies.

Flaxseed oil: It has a very low smoke point, so should not be used in cooking over fire. It is a good choice to be used in salads and salsas.

MCT oil: Medium-chain triglyceride (MCT) oil is most commonly extracted from coconut oil. It is low in calories and an excellent source of energy. Many people enjoy this oil as a salad dressing.

Grapeseed oil: It is extracted from grape seeds. It is high in polyunsaturated fats, which makes it an extremely healthy option. It is a good choice for frying.

Black sesame oil: It is an excellent source of vitamin E and minerals such as copper, iron, zinc, magnesium and calcium. It is used for stir-frying and making pickles.

Pumpkin seed oil: It is lovely for salad dressing, marinades and toppings. It is said to prevent hair loss, ease menopausal symptoms, improve prostate and heart health, and treat an overactive bladder.

Walnut oil: While there are two types of walnut oil available—cold-pressed and refined—you want to focus on the former. Cold-pressed organic walnut oil consists of most of the nutrients that are important for our health.

Coconut oil: This oil is an Indian favourite. It is, however, very high in saturated fats (nearly 90 per cent). Lots of people swear by it, but research has confirmed that we should all stay away from hydrogenated coconut oil. The process of hydrogenation renders the oil, and hence your blood, more viscous, and makes the heart work harder. Coconut oil, however, has a beneficial effect on HDL levels. It has a medium smoking point and is best for low-heat baking and sautéing.

Palm oil: This, too, has a high saturated-fat content, which can be harmful to your heart.

Avocado oil: Almost 70 per cent of avocado oil consists of oleic acid, a monounsaturated omega-9 fatty acid, which is healthy for the heart. It has a high smoke point so it's ideal for baking. You can also drizzle it over soup and while roasting vegetables.

Groundnut oil: Also known as peanut oil, it has a good combination of fats. It has good monounsaturated and polyunsaturated fats and is low in bad saturated fats. It's a good all-purpose oil for cooking.

Mustard oil: This oil has a near-ideal fat composition but is not very good for us, as it contains high amounts of erucic acid, which is known to cause heart problems. Don't use mustard oil as the sole cooking medium. However, it has a high smoking point, so it's very good for deep-frying.

Vegetable oil: Vegetable oil is something most experts don't recommend. Cooking with any sort of vegetable oil releases toxic chemicals linked to cancer and other diseases, according to leading scientists.[2] Vegetable oils are usually extracted at oil mills from soya, corn, sunflower and safflower, and then purified, refined and sometimes chemically altered. It is the chemical treatment that makes vegetable oil unhealthy.

Grow and Eat

If you have any open space at home, even it's very small, I encourage you to grow some food that you are likely to eat every day. It could be herbs such as curry leaves, coriander or even spinach. Some people even grow tomatoes and chillies in pots at home. The joy you will feel when you pluck the food you have so lovingly grown and make it part of your everyday cooking is unparalleled. I know someone whose five-year-old son loves *bhindi* (ladies' finger). He asks for bhindi to be cooked almost every day. So she decided to grow some in her balcony. Now the plant has grown big enough for it to yield seven to eight pieces of bhindi twice a week. That is enough to feed her son. It makes her so happy

---

2   Yue Xin et al, 'Vegetable Oil Intake and Breast Cancer Risk: A Meta-Analysis', *Asian Pacific Journal of Cancer Prevention*, 2015, https://pubmed.ncbi.nlm.nih.gov/26163654/ (accessed on 2 August 2020).

that her son is eating a clean vegetable that she has nurtured. So start small, and soon you'll see the rewards every day.

Choosing What to Eat

Now that we have ensured you've got the best produce, let's have a look at what you can do with it. Studies have shown that eating five or more servings of fruits and vegetables a day can decrease the risk of stroke by 26 per cent, as well as reduce the chance of cardiovascular disease.[3] The more fruits and vegetables you consume, the better it is for your body. But it can be difficult to consume more than the recommended five or more servings in one day, because they do keep us fuller for longer. Other than eating them raw, juicing or blending fruits and vegetables into smoothies are two of the best ways to incorporate them in your diet, which also gives your digestive system rest.

I like all sorts of juices, because they are absorbed into our system in just twenty minutes and start doing their work. Juicing your fruits and veggies ensures that 99 per cent of it is absorbed by the body. Smoothies help me recharge quickly. But be careful, and don't consume packaged juices. No matter what the package tells you, all ready-made juices are sweeter than the ones we make at home. Since I eat clean and simple, my palate is very sensitive. So if there is more of anything in the food, I immediately notice it—salt, sugar or spices. That is why I am sure there must be some hidden

---

[3] Mitra Hariri et al, 'Intakes of Vegetables and Fruits are Negatively Correlated with Risk of Stroke in Iran', *International Journal of Preventive Medicine*, 2013, https://www.ncbi.nlm.nih.gov/pmc/articles/PMC3678236/ (accessed on 2 August 2020).

sugar or preservative in packaged juices even when they say there is nothing added to it. It is best to make juices at home. Juice your fruits and consume them within an hour. Juices are ideal when you are low on energy or before a workout.

Have fresh vegetable juice with breakfast and between meals. And have a turmeric-and-lime shot post your meals. It'll also help you feel active throughout the day. I prefer my juices with more veggies than fruits. The green juice that I had mentioned in the chapter on diets, along with half an avocado, fills me up for dinner. The juice is so good that even twelve hours later, when I get ready for my workout in the morning, I have plenty of energy. In fact, juicing has led to me doing intermittent fasting without even realizing it!

Blending is also an option. The difference between juicing and blending lies in the nutrients left out of the process. With juicing, you're essentially removing all fibrous materials, leaving only the liquid of the fruits and vegetables. With blending, you get it all—the pulp and fibre that bulk up the produce.

Ideally, smoothies should have more fruits and are good for people who don't like to eat veggies. The best benefit of juicing or blending is that they are excellent for digestion. During the process of digestion, food is turned into liquid. When you have nutritious vegetables and fruits in the form of a juice or a smoothie, it's already in liquid form, so your body doesn't have to work hard to digest it, leaving you fresher and less tired.

I would also recommend including as many superfoods in your everyday meals as possible. Superfoods have been given the name for a reason. Superfoods are foods—mostly plant-based—that are thought to be nutritionally dense and thus good for our health. They have many beneficial properties such as antioxidants, which are thought to ward off cancer. They also have healthy fats, which are known to prevent heart disease and fibre, which keeps diabetes and digestive problems at bay.

Goji berries, microalgae, aloe vera, cacao and hemp are some of the superfoods I incorporate into my diet. Goji berries are a good source of vitamins A and C, fibre, iron, zinc and antioxidants. Microalgae are tiny photosynthetic plants that are able to turn energy from the sun into sugars and proteins, absorbing and converting carbon dioxide in the process and expelling oxygen. The most widely known algae are spirulina, chlorella and the blue-green algae AFA. Spirulina is rich in B complex vitamins, vitamin E, iron, calcium, potassium, manganese, zinc, copper and selenium. It is also composed of 60–70 per cent protein and contains essential amino acids, making it a great plant-based protein source. Chlorella is rich in many antioxidants as well, such as vitamins A, C and E, beta-carotene and lutein. It is known to contain more chlorophyll per gram than any other plant. That makes it the ideal food to assist in cleansing and elimination systems, in particular the gut, liver and blood. Blue-green algae is a source of B vitamins, antioxidant compounds and amino acids, along with omega-3 fatty acids. One of its unique nutrients is phenethylamine, which helps in improving one's mood. Microalgae is available in tablet or powder form.

I also consume aloe vera juice, which contains aloe polysaccharides for a healthy digestive system. It helps detoxify the digestive system and assists normal bowel function. Cacao—the dried seeds at the root of chocolate—is also one of the highest sources of magnesium in nature, full of antioxidants, calcium, zinc, copper and selenium.

People consume it in powdered form, mixed with nut milk or yoghurt. Cacao contains more antioxidants per gram than blueberries, goji berries, red wine, raisins, prunes and even pomegranates.

While you're focusing on superfoods, don't forget about superherbs, as they provide an extra boost of nourishment. Ashwagandha, holy basil, shilajit, passion flower, turmeric and ginger are some Ayurvedic superherbs. Turmeric is intensely anti-inflammatory and packed with antioxidants, while ginger decreases muscle soreness caused by intense workouts, calms an upset stomach and helps with motion sickness. Ashwagandha, consumed as a herbal powder, is known to reduce blood sugar levels and stress and anxiety. Tulsi helps manage chronic stress and diabetes, while passion flower relieves insomnia and anxiety. Shilajit, which is available in the form of a powder and capsules, functions as an antioxidant to improve the body's immunity and memory, an anti-inflammatory, an energy booster and a diuretic to remove excess fluid from the body.

Nettles, horse tail, ginseng and lion's mane are some superherbs that originate from outside India. Tea made from nettle leaves is said to reduce inflammation, treat hay fever and lower blood pressure. The horsetail plant, which, like nettle, can be consumed as tea, improves the condition of skin and nails, helps one lose weight by eliminating fluids and strengthens one's bones and tendons. Ginseng is a Chinese superherb, available in extract, capsule or powder form, that reduces inflammation and boosts the immune system. It also gives you energy and lowers blood sugar. The lion's mane mushroom, which is usually sautéed before eating, protects against dementia, reduces mild symptoms of anxiety and depression, and helps repair nerve damage.

Mushrooms are a big source of vitamin D. So if you don't like to go out into the sun, consume mushrooms instead.

Be Smart

While it is important to use these superfoods and superherbs in your everyday diet, what is even more important is where you source them from. A few months ago, I had to travel outside of Mumbai and my son was at home by himself without any help. I was worried about what he would eat for his meals. It's every mother's concern, isn't it? I found a healthy *dabba* service that quoted an extravagant amount. For that much money, they should have been ready with answers to all my questions about how they cooked and where they sourced their meat and vegetables from. But the person I spoke to didn't have a clue. He told me all the vegetables were organic, but didn't know the farms they were bought from. In an attempt to impress me, he also mentioned that a lot of their vegetables were imported and gave me the names of a few countries. Far from being impressed, I had to stop myself from giving him a lecture on the importance of buying local. It's not healthy to eat food that has travelled such long distances. That foodstuff must have lost half of its nutrients on the way. The farther away your food comes from, the worse it is. Imported foods are three times more likely to be contaminated with pathogens than domestic produce. Imported foods, especially fruits and vegetables, often have added chemicals to prevent them from ripening, along with artificial flavour or colour to make them look fresh. A lot of such food is rejected by the strict norms of those countries and hence it all comes to India, where the quality markers are lax. There are so many similar businesses around, which means there are many takers of imported fruits and vegetables. I am, however, not interested in that. I want local, seasonal produce that is grown near my city. That way, I know that the fruits and veggies are as fresh as they can be. Switch from supermarkets to farmer's markets and see how well it reflects in your general well-being.

Eating local is one of the hallmarks of Blue Zones. Blue Zones are places where the local population has better longevity. They all have a few common qualities.

- A cultural environment that reinforces healthy lifestyle habits such as diet and exercise.
- Healthy social relationships and psychological well-being.
- People who have a cooperative spirit.
- People who tend to gardens.
- Public healthcare that is easily accessible.
- Seniors as valued members of the family and the community.

Okinawa in Japan tops the Blue Zone list. It has the world's highest prevalence of proven centenarians—740 out of a population of 1.3 million. Okinawan seniors not only have the highest life expectancy in the world, but also the highest health expectancy. They remain vigorous and healthy far into old age, suffering relatively few age-related ailments. They also follow an old adage that says you should eat until you are 80 per cent full instead of reaching the point where you can't eat any more. It helps you perfect the art of portion control.

One of the best pieces of advice I have to give is that we should all eat the way our grandparents did. They would have moderate portions, practise discipline when it came to food, eat on time and never eat junk food. With a few changes in our diet, we can easily live like our grandparents.

Indians are traditionally known for their home-cooked food. That is why when guests visit us, we prefer to serve them food we've cooked rather than just ordering from outside. It's our way of showing love and care.

I always encourage home cooking. When we go to a restaurant, the food may look prettier than it did at home, but we don't know what has gone into having that plate on our table. We don't know where the ingredients have come from, what oil has been used, if the ingredients were washed with water, if the chefs cleaned their hands thoroughly and used clean vessels. What if the chef was angry because he or she had had a bad day, and they transferred some of that negative energy into the food? Vitamin Love is the best part of home cooking. That's why the food our mothers cook—and, in my case, also that which my husband cooks—tastes so delicious. Why deprive yourself of that love for a cheap imitation?

Organizing Your Pantry

The key to eating healthy is to always be prepared. If your pantry and fridge are stocked with lots of healthy, easy food options, you'll be a lot less likely to order in. Here are some tips you can use to organize your pantry, so home-cooked food is not just an option but your everyday choice:

1. Throw away or donate all food items that don't align with your goal to cook more at home. All processed and ready-to-eat meals should be junked. Keep it if it was grown on a plant and not made in a plant.
2. Stock up the pantry with dry staples such as black-eyed beans, rajma, quinoa, lentils and chia seeds, which you can always have on hand for quick meal options when you're running low on groceries.
3. Stock up on vegetables such as sweet potato, cabbage, beet and carrot because they have a long shelf life—two to three months in the fridge and five weeks outside. That way you always have a healthy starchy option on your hands.
4. Reorganize your fridge to make healthy ingredients easier to find.
5. A good blender or food processor can make all the difference between delicious, nutrient-rich soups, sauces and dips, and inedible food.
6. Keep organic dark chocolate around for a sweet treat. Even a small piece will help curb your sweet cravings without overdoing it. You can also eat a bit of organic jaggery if you want to eat something sweet.

Reading Food Labels

Despite all the processed food we consume these days, we don't know what we're putting into our bodies. We need to read the labels on the back of the box to know that. But reading labels can be tricky. That is because food manufacturers use misleading names to convince us to buy highly processed and unhealthy products. They are also quite difficult to understand. My advice is that if you don't understand something on the label, it is wise to not consume it. I've tried to decode the common things you should look out for when you are purchasing a food item:

1. Product ingredients are listed by quantity—from the highest to lowest as per amounts. This means that the first ingredient is what the manufacturer has used the most. I always check the first three ingredients on the list. If they include refined grains, any type of sugar or hydrogenated oils, I know that the food in the packet is unhealthy.

2. If that packet says 'whole grain', it doesn't mean it is healthy. There are a lot of products that say 'whole grain' on the front, but contain ingredients such as enriched wheat flour or wheat flour. To make enriched wheat flour, all the nutrients in the whole grain are stripped during processing, and synthetic vitamins are added. Similarly, wheat flour does not contain the nutrients that are found in whole wheat—and it is also stripped of its nutrients. Instead, reach for food that has 'whole wheat' or 'unbleached whole wheat' on the label.

3. Don't confuse 'natural' and 'organic' with 'healthy'. Being natural doesn't mean that something is good for you. Organic processed foods such as cookies, granola bars, cereal and muffins aren't any better than regular processed food. It's just processed junk food that probably has a little less of some chemicals.

4. Manufacturers add many types of sugar to hide the actual amount. That way, they can list a healthier ingredient at the top and mention sugar further down the list. They also use different terms to describe sugar to confuse us. Look out for the following names of sugar in the ingredients list: beet sugar, brown sugar, buttered sugar, cane sugar, caster sugar, coconut sugar, date sugar, golden sugar, invert sugar, muscovado sugar, organic raw sugar, rapadura sugar, evaporated cane juice and confectioner's sugar.

    Stevia, erythritol, xylitol, yacon syrup, agave and brown sugar are healthy sugars.

    Types of syrup to be avoided: carob syrup, golden syrup, high-fructose corn syrup, honey, agave nectar, malt syrup, maple syrup, oat syrup, rice bran syrup, and rice syrup.

5. Other added sugars to be avoided include barley malt, molasses, cane-juice crystals, lactose, corn sweetener, crystalline fructose, dextran, malt powder, ethyl maltol, fructose, fruit-juice concentrate, galactose, glucose, disaccharides, maltodextrin and maltose. When the ingredients list says it contains 0 g trans fat but includes partially hydrogenated oil, it means the food contains some trans fat, but less than 0.5 grams per serving. So if

you eat more than one serving, you could end up eating too much trans fat.

6. Pay attention to the calories per serving and how many calories you're actually consuming if you eat the whole packet.

What I Eat

My meals consist of simple, Indian food cooked at home. I am almost a vegetarian, with a rare urge to eat some eggs or organic chicken or fish.

Breakfast

- Fruit of the season.
- Nuts such as walnuts and almonds.
- Seeds such as flax, sunflower and sesame.
- Idli or oats/muesli.
- On rare occasions, I feel like having egg, so I have a masala omelette, a half-boiled or a full-boiled egg. I ensure they are free-range eggs. I have this with multigrain or sourdough toast with organic peanut butter and honey.

Lunch and dinner

- I love all vegetables without exception, so there is plenty for me to choose from. But I am partial to *tendli* (ivy gourd), *doodhi* (bottle gourd), *baingan bharta* (eggplant mash), French beans, carrots, bhindi and mushrooms. All the curries are cooked in minimum oil— sometimes it's just a spray of oil. They are all cooked in only home-ground masalas and with a healthy amount of turmeric. I'm fond of coconut, so a couple of times a week, my sabzis have either coconut milk or grated coconut mixed inside.

- I also love lentils, so the dal is made from different lentils every day.
- Rotis are made from a mixture of all flours, such as bajra, emmer, nachni, ragi, hemp and a minimum amount of wheat flour.
- I have a bowl of salad with any leaves that are available that day and a few slices of grapefruit or pomelo added to it. I don't like salad dressings, so I just season them with a bit of salt and pepper and sour lime. I also add seeds such as flax and sunflower to my salad.
- I have various kinds of sprouts every alternate day.
- I have a small bowl of tomato/spinach/pumpkin soup half an hour before dinner, with a sprinkling of moringa powder.
- I love yams, such as sweet potato, suran and purple yam. I have a portion of boiled sweet potato with chaat masala every day

Evening snack

- A small cup of lactose-free tea or unsweetened almond milk tea with organic peanut butter and sourdough, multigrain or seed toast.

- Makhana, or non-buttered popcorn, when I'm binge-watching a show.

Sweet substitutes

- I don't have chocolate, cake or any kind of dessert. That's also because I don't have a sweet tooth. So if I do want something sweet, I have a couple of dates or dried figs, flavoured yoghurt or low-fat ice cream.

Liquids

- I have coconut water, a nimbu shot or nimbu pani and *kadha* (made with tulsi, ginger, turmeric, licorice, cinnamon, black pepper and cloves) every day. I also drink one litre of alkaline water every day; I add aloe vera pulp juice, chia seeds and two teaspoons of extra-virgin coconut oil to water.

How to Learn Cooking

I'm a lucky girl, because people around me, especially my husband, cook for me. My daughter learnt to cook during college and my son during the lockdown. While I have them, others have parents, siblings, children or cooks to make food for them at home. If you want to start learning to cook on your own, I suggest you look up simple recipes on YouTube. That's a good way to begin. Keep it simple and don't attempt the complicated recipes early on. If you fail, it may put you off cooking. I also recommend checking that you have all your ingredients ready, so you don't get frazzled looking for something in the refrigerator while the pan is on the stove. And, finally, commit to practising cooking regularly. That's the only way to get better at anything—including cooking healthy food at home.

CREATIVITY

Creativity is therapy for the soul.

My father-in-law was one of the most wonderful men anyone could meet. Dr Sharad Panday was one of India's leading cardiac surgeons. Despite his extremely stressful profession, he was a jovial and happy person. I believe a large part of his sunshine personality was thanks to his creative exploits, and his effort and ability to find beauty in the mundane.

He wanted to be an architect when he was a young student, but his parents were keen on their intelligent and brilliant son pursuing a career in cardiac surgery. So that's what he did. But he didn't let his interest in architecture wane. He took an active part in designing our home and his clinic. He also had a green thumb and loved tending to the plants in our garden. However, one of his most endearing quirks was his penchant for collecting anything in the shape of a heart. Whether it was a cup or a mug or a painting or a sculpture, he loved them all and arranged them so beautifully around the home and the clinic. It was this ability to find happiness in simple things that added so much to his life. He didn't chase the things that made the world happy;

he chased what made him happy—his heart in hearts. And that is something most people fail to do.

His creativity was one of the many reasons we got along like a house on fire. Though I am now a fitness professional, I have a degree in commercial art. He and I would have long conversations about art, and I would always feel nourished to my soul after these interactions.

I inherited my creative streak from my father. He worked for an ad agency called Hindustan Lever, and was a well-respected and popular figure throughout the ad world in Asia. In fact, my father was the first person in Asia to start etching on thermocol. He also made paper sculptures and 3D models of products that the company would advertise—all by hand. He was a packaging expert as well and held exhibitions of his creations at Pragati Maidan in Delhi. The best product packaging design at that time was made by my father. My siblings and I grew up watching him create these wonders. There was nobody like him. He knew the importance of his work and creativity in his life, and instilled that in us too. We were always encouraged to explore our artistic sides, even though only I went on to get a formal education in the creative arts.

I, however, later moved into fitness because that was my passion and it was where I knew I belonged. But I have not completely neglected my creative side either. While I would paint in college and gift my work to friends on birthdays, I now use my artistic abilities to design my home and my former gym, Play. About six years ago, when we decided to rebuild our home, I used the wonderful opportunity to get creative. For me, it was a way to pay respect to my father-in-law's legacy. I wanted to refurbish and renovate the house he had set up. Along with our architect, I picked out everything—from the tiles to the paint. In fact, one of my decisions—to use black paint extensively across our home—was unheard of at that time. But the colour looks beautiful on our walls, and we have received so many compliments for it. I did the same for my gym, Play. From choosing the colours of the walls to changing those on the equipment and the layout, I was involved in every decision. The gym looked like one big, beautiful painting, and I am so proud of the creative, fun place I helped create. I like to use some of what I learnt in my degree in my work and surroundings.

I also make sure to write blogs for my website regularly. Even writing this book is a creative outlet for me. As much as I love fitness, I find time to stimulate my creative side once in a while. Creativity has great power in that it allows you to stop and reflect on the things around you and within you. It allows you to express that reflection through the medium of your choice and becomes a living, breathing representation of your thoughts and feelings at the time. It always feels so good to create something. It won't be wrong to say that creativity runs in the Panday family. My husband makes beautiful Ganesha paintings and is an excellent cook; my daughter explores her creative side through fashion; and my son finds joy in acting performances and film. While all of us have other careers, we have balanced them with our creative pursuits. That's probably why none of us suffer from stress. Just like my father-in-law, we, too, have found a way to offset any stress that life can bring by making creativity an important aspect of our lives.

It's not just my family who has done that. When my friend Bipasha Basu noticed that her husband, actor Karan Singh Grover, would doodle on scraps of paper in his free time, she encouraged him to explore his artistic side further.

Karan is already an artiste, albeit a performing one, as one of India's best-known television actors. But those scraps of paper have now morphed into life-size paintings. And Karan's art is so good that he was even invited to display them professionally by a prominent art gallery in Mumbai.

I have witnessed the power of creativity in Karan's transformation from a part-time home doodler to a legitimate, celebrated artist. Similarly, actor Salman Khan paints beautifully with charcoal on canvas, and has auctioned his work for charity. My son too is extremely creative. Whether it is learning how to play the keyboard and guitar, painting or cooking, whatever creative hobby he pursues, he picks up in a matter of days. He is also a beautiful writer and makes his own short films. In fact, he wrote his first film, called *50*, when he was much younger, where he was also the actor and director. He also sings and dances well.

Pour Your Heart Out

Creativity means using your imagination or ideas to create something. In fact, creative ideas don't even have to be original. Sometimes, people build on an existing idea and find a new solution to a current situation. Creative energy is a powerful force. It has the power to transform lives and bring about revolutions. Being creative gives us opportunities to try out new ideas, and new ways of thinking and problem-solving. It helps us acknowledge and celebrate our own uniqueness and diversity. When we tap into our creativity, we are encouraged to express and find ways to create something from personal feelings and experiences. Creativity doesn't necessarily mean you have to draw, paint or create something. It could be the act of making beautiful music on an instrument, writing poetry or even a movie plot, crocheting, knitting, or baking and decorating cakes.

When we think of wellness and good health, we immediately think of diet and exercise. Yes, they are extremely important. But creativity is an overlooked aspect of our overall well-being. Researchers believe that for a well-rounded and healthy lifestyle, one of the neglected aspects is finding that elusive creative outlet.

I have always believed that having projects or hobbies to work on gives us a sense of purpose above and beyond our everyday responsibilities. But now there is scientific research to back that thought up. A 2010 review published in the *American Journal of Public Health* measured how creative practices enhanced health and well-being. Its findings revealed a strong connection between art, and mental and physical health. They found out how creativity led to better mood, decreased anxiety, heightened cognitive function, reduced risk of chronic illnesses and improved immune health.[1]

The Benefits of Creativity

Boosts mood: Ask some of the creative people in your life why they pursue a hobby, and they are likely to say that it is because it makes them feel good. It is something they look forward to outside of their routine. Dedicating part of

---

[1] Heather L. Stuckey and Jeremy Nobel, 'The Connection between Art, Healing, and Public Health: A Review of Current Literature', *American Journal of Public Health*, 2010, https://www.ncbi.nlm. nih.gov/pmc/articles/PMC2804629/ (accessed on 2 August 2020).

your time to something you enjoy is fulfilling and uplifting. You can even turn to it for solace when you've had a bad day. But most of all, it helps build a positive self-identity. When you have a better sense of fulfilment, you are better able to meet your needs and those of the people around you. Repetitive creative hobbies such as knitting, drawing or writing are all tasks that are driven towards results. And when you succeed at something and witness the result, your brain is flooded with dopamine, the feel-good chemical that motivates you to do better.

Reduces anxiety: Research has found that music therapy and theatre are good ways to decrease anxiety.[2] Music calms brain activity and leads to a sense of emotional balance. For people recovering from trauma, writing down their thoughts helps them work out their feelings. With the help of painting or sculpting, a person can use storytelling and imagery to process traumatic events when they find it difficult to put them into words. The average person has about 60,000 thoughts in a day. A creative act can help focus the mind in a way akin to meditation because it calms the brain and the body. We live in stressful times, where our minds are constantly on the move without a moment of rest. Even a little creativity can help you cope with the vagaries of modern life.

---

2   Xi-Jing Chen, Niels Hannibal and Christian Gold, 'Randomized Trial of Group Music Therapy with Chinese Prisoners: Impact on Anxiety, Depression, and Self-Esteem', *International Journal of Offender Therapy and Comparative Criminology*, 2015, https://journals.sagepub.com/doi/abs/10.1177/0306624X15572795 (accessed on 2 August 2020).

Boosts brain function: Researchers have also found that creativity has an immense positive impact on the brain. Musicians have been studied for a heightened connectivity between their left and right brain hemispheres. Einstein, too, was an excellent violinist, and this possibly helped him effectively use both sides of his brain simultaneously. Working on something creative, whether it's writing a story, tending a garden or cooking, helps apply problem-solving and critical-thinking skills. Creativity will always come to use when you face inevitable obstacles and challenges in life. When we make creativity a habit, we continue to learn and inculcate resourceful ways of solving problems.

Creativity is also an effective treatment for patients with dementia. Studies have shown that indulging in creative acts not only reduces depression and isolation, but can also help people with dementia tap into their personalities and sharpen their senses.[3]

Increases immunity: Studies have looked at how music helps restore the health of the immune system and decreases the body's response to inflammation, which is a root cause of many illnesses.[4] People who journal their experiences every day actually have stronger immune-

---

[3] Beat Ted Hannemann, 'Creativity with Dementia Patients', *Gerontology*, 2006, https://lemosandcrane.co.uk/resources/Gerontology%20-%20Creativity%20with%20Dementia%20Patients.pdf (accessed on 2 August 2020).

[4] Daisy Fancourt, Adam Ockelford and Abi Abebech Belai, 'The Psychoneuroimmunological Effects of Music: A Systematic Review and A New Model', *Brain Behavior and Immunity*, 2013, https://www.researchgate.net/publication/258042912_The_Psychoneuroimmunological_Effects_of_Music_A_Systematic_Review_and_A_New_Model (accessed on 2 August 2020).

system function. Writing increases your CD4+ lymphocyte count, the key to the immune system. For people with existing chronic illnesses, having a creative outlet can also help in the healing process by reducing stress hormones and inflammation.[5] When you set aside time to create for your own pleasure, it relieves whatever stress and tension you've been under.

Leads to a sense of pride: Knowing that you are responsible for creating something and letting other people know about it is a wonderful feeling. I know someone who attended a painting class once, even though she was a self-confessed non-creative person. She wasn't good at painting or drawing, but by following the instructions in the painting class, she created something beautiful that she wouldn't have been able to before the class. Now that painting holds price of place in her living room, a testament that all of us can be good at a lot of things we are sure we won't succeed at.

Creativity allows us to depict how we perceive our world. Expressing yourself through a canvas or a piece of music is an uplifting feeling that brings forth individuality like nothing else, and also leaves part of you behind for others to enjoy and benefit from.

Unlike most societal pursuits, creative pursuits are free-flowing. They have no strict guidelines. It's always a comma, never a full stop. There's always more to do.

---

5   Keith J. Petrie et al, 'Effect of Written Emotional Expression on Immune Function in Patients with Human Immunodeficiency Virus Infection: A Randomized Trial', *Psychosomatic Medicine*, 2004, https://pubmed.ncbi.nlm.nih.gov/15039514/ (accessed on 2 August 2020).

Nothing is right, nothing is wrong—and this infinite depth is what makes it so unique and fulfilling.

How to Find Your Creative Side

Start small: When we compare our creativity to others', we may feel like we are incapable of being as good as they are. But the point of indulging in any type of creative activity, especially when it's not your means of income, is to just have fun while doing it and not worry about the results. Why not start small and see how you feel about it after giving it a shot? This small change will become an enjoyable habit. Here are some ideas for you to take that first step to explore your creative side:

- Play around with your wardrobe by wearing tops and bottoms you've never worn together. Notice how you feel. Challenge yourself to wear a new combination of clothes each day of the week.
- Sort through old clutter, find better ways to utilize your space, or try hanging something new on a wall in your home. Not only will you tap into your creative side, but you'll also end up with tidier and prettier surroundings.
- Start writing, and don't stop until you've reached 500 words. Write down anything that comes to mind.
- Write in a journal while listening to three different types of music on three different days and see how you feel. Do certain types of music affect your mood in any particular way? Did your writing style change according to the music?

- Write a poem in emojis and see if a friend or a family member can understand it.
- Change your bathroom routine by brushing your teeth with your non-dominant hand.
- Invent a new sandwich. What ingredients would you use? What would you call it? What would be your secret ingredient to set this sandwich apart from others?

Listen to your heart and follow it blindly. When my son was eight and *Dhoom 2* had released, he went around doing the iconic whistle step in front of everyone he saw. I would observe how people would look at him for only the first one minute and then look away, but he wouldn't stop. He did it because it gave him joy, not for other people's reactions. Similarly, your creative pursuits shouldn't be based on what others think of it. It should be driven by how it makes you feel. To make sure you don't leave a creative exercise midway, there are some things you can do:

Try different things: Figure out what you enjoy. You could like to write poems or short stories, dance, paint, crochet, take photographs, cook or design your home. It could be something else too. The point is to enjoy it. But you'll never find out if you don't try. My son tries everything that piques his interest. He enjoys every bit of learning something new and becomes a master at it before moving on to something new.

Partner up with someone: A lot of times we tend to feel bored when it's just us doing an activity. Ask a friend or one of your parents to do it with you. It could be a great way to spend time with each other, work on your relationships and also have fun in the process.

Be open to new experiences: You will learn plenty from doing something as simple as taking a new route home from work or seeking out a new group of people with different interests.

Schedule some creative time: I'd also recommend carving out space in your home where you can work on your creative projects. Keep a journal of ideas that inspires creativity and write them down as they come to you. And, of course, schedule your creative time into your calendar and treat it as a priority.

Exercises to Cultivate Creativity

A large part of creativity is about thinking outside the box. There are some exercises you can do to tap into your creativity and use your mind in different ways. These exercises can help broaden the horizons of your mind and increase problem-solving skills.

1. A major benefit of cultivating creativity is to view issues and problems as opportunities for innovation, growth and improvement. Spend fifteen minutes walking around your home or office, and write down ten issues that catch your attention. Then spend ten minutes brainstorming one solution to each problem. For instance, if you are bored with the furniture set-up of your home but don't have money to redecorate, a possible solution could be to rearrange the furniture to give the room new energy.

2. Now take one problem from your personal life and write down as many solutions to the problem you can think of. For instance, if you're working late on the same day that your friends are coming over for dinner and you don't have time to prepare a three-course meal, what do you do? Maybe you can order in some of the food and cook the rest, or you can ask if the project deadline can be extended by a day.

3. A study featured in the *Personality and Social Psychology Bulletin* shows that when people are thinking and creating on behalf of someone else, they are more innovative than when they are building something for themselves. So imagine your supervisor has asked you to organize a work party. What would you do? Where would you go? What sort of food would you have? What would be the main activities at the party? What sort of music would you play? Write down as many details about this party as possible.

Creativity at the Workplace

Just as in your personal life, being creative at work has its benefits.

Better team work and bonding: Creative team-building activities at work have been proven to be beneficial. Since most forms of creativity are not competitive, you and your colleagues are unlikely to bring rivalry into the mix and work together as a team.

Better morale: Being creative makes people happy. If your colleagues are happy, you are happy, and everyone will work better and be more productive. As stated in *Harvard Business Review*: 'There is nothing more satisfying that watching your people fulfil the human need to create and having their creative contributions benefit the organisation and the markets it serves.'[6]

Organizational growth: Creativity is about the opportunity to see, make or do something new. Reports have shown that organizations that work towards showing, making or doing something new are the ones that survive.

It's plain for everyone to see that being creative makes you happy and stress-free. By doing so, you create balance

---

[6]   Ron Carucci, 'How to Nourish Your Team's Creativity', *Harvard Business Review*, May 2017, https://hbr.org/2017/05/how-to-nourish-your-teams-creativity (accessed on 2 August 2020).

in your circle of life, which is what I wish for everyone to have. A creative life is an amplified life, so why deny yourself that chance? Also, there's no harm in having a few tricks up your sleeve. You never know what opportunity may come your way to showcase a skill.

EDUCATION

Sometimes you win, sometimes you learn.

One day I was waiting to hail an autorickshaw, when a sophisticated-looking man passed me. He was talking on the phone in crisp diction and I overheard him talking about the 17-kilometre run he went on that morning. A well-spoken man talking about fitness! I smiled to myself, glad to see someone taking care of themselves. But the pleasant feeling didn't last long. A few paces after he had crossed me, the man spat on the footpath before continuing his conversation on the phone.

I couldn't believe what I had just seen. He was clearly educated and should have known better than to spit in a public place. But he was just one on a long list of people who don't have the right moral and civic values, despite access to the best things in life. After having met many such people, I have realized that they are merely literate—they aren't educated. They can read and write, with some having attended some of the finest schools and colleges, but they haven't learnt much.

Good education means putting the knowledge you have to good use. Otherwise, all you have is a bunch of concepts and no idea how to apply them to your everyday life.

Literacy is the ability to read and write, whereas education is being able to understand fundamental concepts and using your skills to improve your own life as well as of those around you. Even a robot can read and write, but using knowledge wisely is what makes humans different.

Education begins for all of us at school. Our teachers and professors teach us what they believe we need to succeed in life. I know all my teachers had good intentions, but I sometimes think back to my school and college days, and remember how much I learnt only by rote. The Indian education system is geared towards making you score high marks and not really arming students with the skills and knowledge they need to navigate life. Education must be preceded by curiosity. When we are curious about something, we try to find out as much as we can about a subject and are eager to educate ourselves. A good educational system should instil a sense of curiosity in students, to help them look beyond what is in a textbook, and also give them the confidence to apply what they learn to everyday life.

Education gives us knowledge of the world and a different perspective of looking at life. It also helps us build opinions. We all know people who may not have degrees but are very aware of what is going on around them. Education is not just about lessons in textbooks—it is about the lessons of life. And when you truly learn to make your life better with it, you make good use of your education.

Benefits of Education

When education is imparted in the correct fashion, it has the power to change the world. Here are a few of its extraordinary benefits:

Promotes equality: Education is one of the greatest equalizers. Equal access to education is necessary so that everyone, regardless of caste, gender or social class, gets equal opportunities to succeed. A lack of education often deprives people of better job or career opportunities. Access to quality education definitely gives marginalized people a chance to improve their means of living.

Economic growth: Countries with high literacy rates have citizens with high per capita incomes. In contrast, developing countries, where a large number of people live below the poverty line, usually have high illiteracy rates. For instance, in 2050, the GDP per capita in low-income countries will be almost 70 per cent lower than it would be if all the children in those countries were educated.[1]

Better health: Children of educated parents have a higher chance of living a healthier life. This is because they are more likely to receive vaccinations, better nourishment, have better access to health facilities and even moral support.

Builds awareness: Blind faith and superstitions have had a devastating effect on Indian society. Education helps us question and analyse the information that is made available to us every day, and be able to determine what is correct and what is not. An educated mind asks for logic and scientific reasoning behind all actions. This is a critical skill for success later in life.

Greater sense of discipline: As students, we learnt how to manage time and create our own success, which also taught

---

[1] https://report.educationcommission.org/ (accessed on 2 August 2020).

us self-discipline. This is such an important aspect of whatever we do, whether it is in work, fitness, diet or financial planning.

Sense of accomplishment: Finishing any degree is an accomplishment that should be celebrated. Graduating gives students a huge sense of achievement and the confidence they need to go out into the world and make something of themselves.

Sense of independence: Education gives you the skills and knowledge to pursue a career that you are interested in, and, in the process, makes you financially secure. Working in a career of your choice, as we have learnt from the chapter on career, is immensely satisfying and gives purpose to your life.

Empowerment: Education helps turn weaknesses into strengths. It gives people the confidence to stand up for themselves and improve their decision-making capabilities. Research has proven that in countries such as India, where women are subjected to gender bias, education helps them tackle marital violence and take charge of their lives.[2] My favourite young achiever, Malala Yousafzai, was shot because she wanted to go to school and educate herself. In her address at the United Nations in 2013, she said, 'Books and our pens, they are the most powerful weapons. One child, one teacher, one

---

2   Bhartiya Stree Shakti, 'Tackling Violence against Women: A Study of State Intervention Measures', Ministry of Women and Child Development, Government of India, 2017, https://wcd.nic.in/sites/default/files/Final%20Draft%20report%20BSS_0.pdf (accessed on 2 August 2020).

book and one pen can change the world. Education is the only solution. Education first.'[3]

Why Homeschooling Is an Excellent Idea

When my kids were growing up, I didn't know much about homeschooling. That was because it wasn't really popular in India a decade ago. However, having read up on it and heard experiences of some people who are currently homeschooling their children, if I had to do it all over again, I would probably opt for homeschooling for my children. During the 2020 lockdown because of the COVID-19 pandemic, parents got the chance to homeschool their kids, and some of my friends, while initially frustrated, spoke about its many benefits.

One-on-one tutoring: Students always benefit from a smaller student-teacher ratio, and what can be better than the 1:1 ratio you can provide at home? Learning at home ensures that children master a skill or a concept, and only then move on to the next topic. It takes away the pressure of studying for an exam and getting marks, and, instead, focuses on learning for the joy of it and using it to keep learning more.

Tailor-made education: Every child is different, and each has his or her varied needs. In such a scenario, every student may not get the customized attention and teaching they need in a school that has more than thirty students in each class. With homeschooling, parents can personalize their child's

---

[3] Malala Yousafzai, '"One Child, One Teacher, One Pen And One Book Can Change The World"', *Outlook*, 10 December 2014, https://www.outlookindia.com/website/story/one-child-one-teacher-one-pen-and-one-book-can-change-the-world/292810 (accessed on 2 August 2020).

education to maximize learning, work on their weaknesses and focus on special areas of the child's interest or talent.

No more boredom: Since learning is specifically tailored, it makes kids put in a more consistent effort into learning. They don't waste time on what they have already learnt while other kids are catching up. Homeschooling removes the stress children undergo these days because of the volume of homework assigned to them. Thanks to homeschooling, learning becomes fun and more engaging.

Better social interactions: With a flexible curriculum, parents can take their children to museums, parks and historical sites in their city. This has shown to improve emotional and psychological development in children. Family connections are also strengthened when students homeschool with their siblings. Kids gain a greater awareness of the world around them and can develop a stronger sense of civic responsibility.

The quality parents will need in abundance when they decide to homeschool is patience—with themselves as well as their kids. There are all sorts of curriculums online and you can choose which one you want to follow according to what you think will benefit your child. You can also take the help of videos online to explain concepts that you have difficulty teaching.

Take a Leaf from Their Book of Life

Whether you choose homeschooling or the traditional institutional way of teaching, the world has shown us that education only goes so far in determining your success. There are so many examples of people who never had degrees from the best colleges in the world but were wildly successful. Apple creator Steve Jobs was one of them. He went to college in the US for just six months, and then dropped out. But he had a great idea for a revolutionary product and he created it with his friend Steve Wozniak. Closer home, Azim Premji also dropped out of Stanford University after completing his graduation from St Xavier's College in Mumbai. But he went on to found Wipro and is now a billionaire.

I don't want to just talk about people who went on to earn a lot of money. There are people such as Arunachalam Muruganantham as well, who invented a simple machine that changed the lives of lakhs of rural women. He didn't have a chance to finish his schooling, but he identified that women in rural areas didn't have access to sanitary pads, and thus made a machine that could produce this essential item at an extremely affordable cost.

This is not to say that only those who haven't completed their education can become successful. Our doctors, engineers, teachers and bankers are all where they are because they educated themselves in a field of their choice and pursued careers that fulfilled them. Whether institutionally educated or not, what matters at the end of the day is that you have a passion to do what you want to. Our mothers make the lip-smacking food they cook because of the love and joy they get from feeding their families. A Le Cordon Bleu chef also does the same, just at a restaurant. What they have in common is their love for food, regardless of whether they went to food school.

Seeking knowledge is a lifelong process. Every day is a new opportunity for you to learn something you didn't know the day before. It doesn't always have to benefit you monetarily for that knowledge to be considered educational. I know someone who works in a bank, but is an aspiring ornithologist. She loves watching birds and takes up every opportunity to learn more about them. She's gaining an education in a field that isn't her career and I'm proud of her for exploring her interests.

Any sort of education has the power to change our mindset and our lives. Education is an integral spoke in our circle of life, because it gives us the opportunity to expand our mindset and explore ideas that we wouldn't have known otherwise. Aim to be educated and not just literate, and see how well it benefits your overall life.

Reading Can Calm You Down

This is one of my favourite reasons for picking up a book to read. A study conducted by the University of Essex, UK, found that reading for just six minutes could reduce stress levels by 60 per cent.[4] Reading slows the heart rate, lowers blood pressure and calms our minds. It is said that losing ourselves in a book is the ultimate relaxation. It really doesn't matter what book we are reading. By losing ourselves in a thoroughly engrossing book, we can escape the worries and stresses of everyday life.

To illustrate how good reading is, some time ago, my son injured his shoulder and was told to recuperate at home. He started reading so much that he would sometimes finish a book in a day. This just shows that sometimes difficult moments lead to beautiful destinations.

---

[4] http://nationalreadingcampaign.ca/wp-content/uploads/2013/09/ReadingFacts1.pdf (accessed on 2 August 2020).

SOCIAL LIFE

Enjoy the way you want to, not how others think you should.

The year 2020 began the same way all new years begin— with hope and a prayer that it will be better than the one that went by. But then the pandemic hit and it became *annus horribilis*. It was initially a bit like a holiday for some people, giving them a chance to catch up on their reading, watch TV shows and movies, and finally learn to cook. But soon things got real. Living a life where we didn't meet anyone other than our families (and sometimes not even them) became the new normal.

While some were feeling like caged animals who couldn't wait to step out, I was content to be at home. My husband and I are both homebodies, since we both work from home and even spend our free time at home. I usually step out only for work-related activities or when my friends and I are celebrating a milestone. So our lives pretty much stayed the same. In fact, thanks to the enforced lockdown, there were some additional advantages, such as considerably less pollution, more birds chirping outside my balcony, dolphins appearing along the Mumbai coast, cleaner beaches and much less noise pollution, along with a sense of calm and serenity that I haven't experienced before in Mumbai. I also finally watched people live the kind of lifestyle I have been advocating for a long time—the slow life. Don't get me wrong, a slow life doesn't mean an unproductive life. In fact, it is meant to be more successful and productive. I'll explain more later in the chapter.

While my husband and I adapted very well to the isolation, there are a few things I missed. I missed going to the gym and the people I met there. I also missed meeting my mother, my siblings and celebrating with my friends. I missed people. But I revelled in spending time with myself and my family, exercising at home and reading. Meditation and yoga helped me find mental peace and calm, so I didn't panic or get anxious about the alarming news of the virus and its devastating impact, which just kept piling up.

My personality type—I am a classic ambivert—also played its part. Ambiverts adapt to change quite well. We mould ourselves to the demands of the situation and aren't inconvenienced by it. Unlike an extrovert, I don't need to be out and about every evening, and unlike an introvert, social situations don't tax me. As an ambivert, I enjoy the company of people as well as of myself. When I am with friends or at a rare party I attend, I enjoy myself thoroughly. And I also love my own company and can sit by myself for hours. I am never bored or anxious of being alone or in the midst of people.

However, at the same time, the situation enforced by the pandemic was really tough on some people. I heard more people around me speak of the anxiety, depression and nightmares they were experiencing because of being cut off from others, and the uncertainty the lockdown and the virus brought. Social isolation can have a huge impact on your mental and physical health, sleep and diet, and increase the risk of depression, anxiety, panic attacks and tiredness and lack of motivation. At such times, meditation can help you get rid of discomforting and unpleasant thoughts.

Why Social Life Matters

Man is a social animal. We aren't built to live in isolation. A healthy social life is necessary for our mental and physical health. Throughout history, humans have spent their life in small groups, where each individual is dependent on others for survival. Those who were separated from their tribe often suffered severe consequences, in the form of early death. That condition of interdependence is what we have all best adapted to. These days, technology has changed the way people interact with others, but it hasn't affected the basic need to have supportive relationships with other people.

My daughter lives and works in Los Angeles. When she had just moved there, she found it a bit difficult to meet people, despite being a friendly person. It took her a few months to find friends she bonded with and whom she could spend time with. Like my daughter, if you've ever moved away from home, you'll have a good idea of just how much your social circle shapes your everyday life. One study showed that the extent of social connection is a greater determinant of health than obesity, smoking and high blood pressure.[1] Along with meeting people, social connection also means feeling understood and connected to others.

---

[1] Ning Xia and Huige Li, 'Loneliness, Social Isolation, and Cardiovascular Health', *Antioxidants and Redox Signaling*,

Good, steady friendships have so much to offer us. They give us a sense of belonging, purpose and happiness, reduce our stress and improve our self-worth and confidence. Research has shown that social connections not only impact your mental health, but your physical health as well. A review of 148 studies shows that people with strong social relationships had a 50 per cent higher chance of longer lives.[2]

Despite the hyper-connectedness of our world, a lot of people are lonely. And it's not always easy to admit to it. When people suppress these feelings, it can often add to depressive and even suicidal thoughts. One study found that loneliness is as bad for your health as smoking fifteen cigarettes a day.[3] When you're happy and your mind is healthy, you are unlikely to feel alone.

The truth is that we need people around us to help us live and enrich our life, not just survive. The last few months notwithstanding, everyone has a social life that they are comfortable with. Everyone falls in three broad categories when we classify them by their social life: extroverts, introverts and ambiverts.

2018, https://www.ncbi.nlm.nih.gov/pmc/articles/PMC5831910/ (accessed on 3 August 2020).

[2] Julianne Holt-Lunstad, Timothy B. Smith and J. Bradley Layton, 'Social Relationships and Mortality Risk: A Meta-Analytic Review', *PLOS Medicine*, 2010, https://journals.plos.org/plosmedicine/article?id=10.1371/journal.pmed.1000316 (accessed on 3 August 2020).

[3] Julianne Holt-Lunstad, 'Testimony before the US Senate Aging Committee', 2017; https://www.aging.senate.gov/imo/media/doc/SCA_Holt_04_27_17.pdf (accessed on 3 August 2020).

Are You an Extrovert?

Extroverts are more easily able to develop their social lives. They attend parties and meetings often, and interact with many people and develop different kinds of relationships with them. Their outgoing nature draws people to them and they have a hard time turning away from attention. They thrive on interactions with people.

In the 1960s, psychologist Carl Jung first described introverts and extroverts when discussing personality elements. He classified these two groups based on where they found their source of energy. Jung said that extroverts were energized by crowds and by interaction with the external world. To know if you are one, check how much you agree with the points below:

- *You enjoy social settings:* People with more extroverted tendencies like being the centre of attention. They actively look forward to being in social situations. They are also not afraid of introducing themselves to new people and rarely avoid unfamiliar situations for fear of not knowing someone.
- *You don't like a lot of alone time:* For extroverts, too much alone time drains their energy. They feel energized in good company.
- *You like large groups:* Extroverts thrive around people and some even take charge of group activities. They rarely turn down invitations to weddings, parties and other gatherings.
- *You make new friends easily:* We all know people who are great at striking up conversations with new people and go on to become good friends

with them. As someone who is the opposite of that, I have always found this quality fascinating. Extroverts enjoy other peoples' energy, and because they pursue new interests and activities, they are often keen to expand their social circles.

- *You prefer to talk out problems:* While introverts tend to internalize problems and think them through, extroverts are willing to express themselves openly and prefer to take their problems to others for guidance.

- *You are optimistic:* Extroverts are often described as happy, positive and cheerful. While they experience difficulties and troubles just like the rest of us, it isn't always easy to make out they are going through a tough time.

- *You aren't afraid of taking risks:* Extroverts are more likely to take risks and experience a rush of dopamine if the risk pays off. This lights up the reward centre of the brain and encourages them to take risks in the future as well.[4]

- *You are flexible:* Extroverts are able to adapt to different situations and get innovative when problems arise. While they may be organized, not all extroverts need a plan of action before they can begin a project, plan a vacation or undertake a task. They take spontaneous decisions.

---

[4] Ronald Fischer, Anna Lee and Machteld N. Verzijden, 'Dopamine Genes Are Linked to Extraversion and Neuroticism Personality Traits, but Only in Demanding Climates', *Scientific Reports*, 2018, https://www.nature.com/articles/s41598-017-18784-y (accessed on 3 August 2020).

Are You an Introvert?

Carl Jung believed that introverts needed alone time to recharge. They are often quieter and more reserved in their manners, personality and engagement with others. They focus on internal thoughts and feelings rather than seek out the company of others. My husband is a textbook introvert. To know if you are one, check how much you agree with the points below:

- *You find people energy-draining:* Do you ever feel exhausted after spending time with a lot of people? Introverts feel the need to retreat to a quiet place or into themselves after interacting with others longer than they'd like. While they do enjoy spending time around others, they prefer the company of close friends.
- *You enjoy solitude:* An introvert's idea of a good time is a quiet afternoon to themselves to enjoy what they like.
- *You have a small group of close friends:* People believe that introverts don't like people because they don't like to socialize. However, they prefer having a small group of close friends to a large social circle.
- *People describe you as quiet:* Introverts are often described as quiet and reserved. They are even mistaken for being shy because of their tendency to choose their words carefully and not waste time on needless chit-chat.
- *You are self-aware:* Because introverts tend to introspect, they also spend a great deal of time

examining their own experiences. They tend to be more self-aware than extroverts because they spend time learning about themselves.

Are You an Ambivert?

Human beings are complex creatures, and we don't always behave the way we are expected to. If you feel like either of the above descriptions don't quite fit you, you could be an ambivert. You display extroverted or introverted behaviour according to the situation. This section speaks to me the most because I am basically describing myself here.

- *You are a good listener and communicator:* Extroverts prefer to talk more, while introverts observe and listen. But ambiverts know when to speak up and when to listen.
- *You like being with people, and yourself:* Ambiverts can equally like being in a crowd or at home. It all depends on their frame of mind.
- *Empathy comes naturally to you:* They are able to listen and understand where a person is coming from. If a friend is having an issue, an extrovert might try to offer a solution right away, and an introvert might be able to listen to the problem, but an ambivert will listen and ask questions so that they can help.
- *You are able to provide balance:* In a group, ambiverts can provide some much-needed balance. For instance, they can be the ones to break an awkward silence and make everyone feel comfortable.

How to Balance Work, Family and Social Life

No one wants to party all the time. Even people who love partying don't want to party all the time. It's the same with work and, yes, even our families. We all need a break from the routine of our life once in a while. People who work long hours don't have much time to meet their friends. This can create distance and lead to resentment and stress in relationships. Spending time with the people we love is something we should all pencil into our timetables. But if you are struggling to do so, here are a few ideas you could adopt without ruining your social life:

- *Go on a vacation:* It's difficult to get leave from work sometimes for a longer vacation, but try to plan a holiday at least once a year with your loved ones. If you are unable to stay away from work for an extended time, try more frequent but shorter getaways. They will be a good break from work. You can also turn weekends into mini-vacations and recharge yourself in the company of friends.
- *Turn a work skill into a personal project:* If you are a great communicator or enjoy planning events, how about extending your work skills to a cause that inspires you? That way you will enjoy performing those tasks and help someone who hasn't had the same opportunity.
- *Socialize with your co-workers:* Create a balance between your work and social life by hanging out with your colleagues. You can also invite them home by throwing a dinner party. You'll also get

to know them outside the workplace and discover wonderful aspects of their personalities.

- *Unplug:* There are times when you should just switch your phone off—or at least disable notifications— and enjoy the moment. Not doing so interrupts your off time and adds an undercurrent of stress. So don't text your boss when you're having dinner with friends, and don't send work emails while you're with family.

- *Start small:* Many workaholics promise their friends and family that they will never attend to work when they are with them. But that isn't always possible. So, instead, pick out a dedicated time for work, and then devote the rest to spending time with them? That will be easier to do as well, and guilt or resentment will not creep in.

How to Build a Social Life

If you find yourself feeling awkward among a group of people, it could affect your social life and sometimes even your career. Connecting with people around us and those we work with contributes to better mental health. Here's how you can find joy in connecting with people.

- When you meet new people, turn the conversation to topics you find comfortable, know enough about and can give you enough to talk about, such as the shows you may have been watching or the last place either of you travelled to. You could even ask them to recommend restaurants in your area. One of the best conversation starters is to ask people about the work they do. Remember to share something about yourself too, so that it's actually a conversation and you don't end up listening to a monologue.

- Be a good listener. It is only when we listen that we learn about people. It could be something cool your colleague is talking about or a confession your friend is trying to make. At the end of the conversation, you will know that person a little more than you did before. Listening is a great way to make new friends and feel closer to people who are already part of your life.

- Learn something new. Join a salsa class or learn to bake from the neighbourhood aunty who is known for her delicious cupcakes. You will end up meeting more people. Once you've become acquaintances, try and spend more time with them if you enjoy their company.

- Check your body language. We all communicate non-verbally as well. The way we conduct ourselves physically impacts how others perceive us. Loosen up, relax, make eye contact and appear open to a conversation.

- Stay away from negative thoughts. If you are one of those people who believes that you are awkward in a social setting and constantly talk about it, no matter how much you work at your social skills, you are unlikely to go too far. Tell yourself that you won't embarrass yourself in a group and that you will smile more and engage in conversation. You don't want the negative talk to become a self-fulfilling prophecy, do you?

Slow Down

The recent self-isolation that large parts of the world went or is going through also brings to mind an important aspect of our social lives—the need to slow down. A lot of us couldn't wait to get out. But a lot of people also found the time to turn to activities that they had put on hold for a long time.

I know of a friend who was grateful that she got some much-needed time for herself. By slowing down, she could spent a lot more time with her daughter and enjoy that relationship more.

This isolation has awakened my friend and many like her to the idea that slowing down is a kind of soft reboot, and we can all learn to enjoy the small joys of life.

I have been living the slow life for many years now. I do my work at my own pace, without the need to hurry up and move to the next thing. I take out time every day to spend with myself, my family and my pets.

I believe that the pandemic has had many lessons for us—one of which is to cherish what we have and understand the true meaning of life. There will always be work, but the precious time we spend with our family and doing things that make our soul sing can help us immensely.

Benefits of Slowing Down

The world we live in is constantly hustling or moving on to the next thing. That keeps our bodies and minds in a constant mode of stress. Slowing down is the opposite of hustling. These days, slowing down can be the difference between success and failure, between thriving and burning out. In fact, slowing down means you are sometimes even more productive than before. Here are a few reasons you should practise it.

- *You'll have greater clarity:* Too many people go endlessly down a path that won't give them the results they want. It's like you running on a treadmill or the hamster running on its wheel—you're working but you're not going anywhere. To change this, schedule an hour every week to check in with yourself. Reflect on your intentions and look for the challenges or opportunities showing up in front of you. Think about what's working and what's not, and where else you can focus your energies.

- *You'll make better decisions:* When you slow down, indulge in self-care and make time for rest, relaxation and meditation, you lower your baseline for mental stress. When your mind isn't racing, it is free to absorb information, assess the situation and take good decisions.

- *You will perform better:* If you can't perform at your optimum level, you can't do your best and create the life you want. If your goal is to succeed, you should take the time to acknowledge what your mind, body and spirit need to stay healthy. When every day gives you twenty-four hours, you have no excuse not to meditate, exercise, cook a healthy meal or keep a journal.

- *You will understand your emotions better:* By slowing down, you can better feel and understand the emotions you're experiencing. That way you can process them and let them guide you to a healthy response. For instance, your anger can tell you a great deal about yourself. It lets you know that something is wrong. When that energy is channelled, it gives you clarity to change the situation. If you are hustling all the time, anger will get the better of you, and you will act on it. The adverse effects can undo your progress and keep you from the success you want. Slowing down helps you turn emotions into actions that then lead you to success.

How to Slow Down

I know a lady who is in her late forties and lives a very busy life. Her work requires her to be in different time zones every few days. She is a workaholic and thrives on it. She also works out compulsively every day, and longer than the one hour most people spend at the gym. That, along with crash diets, has given her an enviable body. She also drinks a lot of coffee to keep up with her hectic life. What she doesn't realize is that soon she will burn out. This kind of lifestyle, where you are constantly on the go, is not sustainable and affects your body and mind in terrible ways. This lady is constantly on a fight-or-flight mode, which is an unhealthy way to live. She believes and loves to show off that she is leading an incredible life, but she is mistaken. In fact, to thrive, she should be living the exact opposite life. What she needs to do is slow down. There are a few ways you can slow down, or at least begin the process so that you keep getting better at it.

- *Choose three things to accomplish every day:* I am sure you can come up with a long list of things you would like to accomplish, but don't. Keeping the list small will force you to decide what's really important. When you finish the list, you can relax for the rest of the day.

- *Learn to say no:* How often have you said yes to something that you haven't wanted to do in the first place? And then you kept grumbling while doing it and couldn't wait for the task to get over? By taking on responsibility that you don't want to or can't manage to fulfil, you will only stretch yourself too thin. Where is the joy in that?
- *Be unproductive but yet productive:* The world has evolved to look down on people who don't do as much as they can. But that is a wrong approach. The race to be productive and to create something all the time is robbing us of happiness and making us robots. Make time every day to just laze around and do what you want to do, instead of what you should do. By doing so, you are freeing up your mind. A free mind is a productive mind, because it is unencumbered by the stresses of life. In fact, it may lead to some great ideas and give you the chance to get creative. So by giving your mind and yourself some time to just chill, you are, in fact, gearing yourself up to be more productive in life.
- *Use social media infrequently:* Mindless scrolling has almost become like an addiction, which steals time you could spend doing stuff that actually makes you happy. So leave that phone behind and take out that dusty list of things you have always wanted to do but never seemed to have had the time for.

- *Find a hobby:* Try something new, even if you aren't going to excel at it. As long as it excites you and taps into your creativity, you will have fun. Try any or all of these—yoga, running, whittling, reading, blogging, gardening, chess and painting.

- *Pause and notice the beauty around you:* I spend a few minutes every day gazing at the peepul tree outside my balcony. I watch the birds that sit on the branches and how the leaves move and change colour as the sunlight hits them. An involuntary smile lights up my face when I see the beauty that's around me. Trees are beautiful, and so is the sky every time you look up at it. You'll love the calm that comes with it.

- *Spend time with people you love:* There is no piece of advice or suggestion better than this. Our family, friends and social circle form the backbone of a purposeful life. Sharing secrets, fears and hopes with another human is the best way to slow down and enjoy life. Without other people, we become lonely beings. Make time for your loved ones, regardless of your personality type. Rely on your social circle and you'll see your life becoming fuller. Identify what kind of personality you are and strike a balance. If you are an extrovert, embrace some qualities of an introvert or an ambivert, and vice versa. That way, you will learn to balance your social life. The people in life—the ones who are close to us and the ones we know only as acquaintances—contribute to our sense of identity. Our lives are better, thanks to our social circle, and there is no substitute for the balance they provide to our life.

Colour to Slow Down

Colouring books for adults have become quite popular over the past few years. They come with beautiful, intricate designs and solution for your mental health. I have been colouring for a while now and I love its many benefits:

- Colouring books reduce stress, as they calm down our amygdala. This is the part of the brain that controls our fight or flight response, and keeps us in a heightened state of worry, panic and hyper-vigilance. Colouring and focusing on this harmless and calming activity can actually turn that response down and let your brain have some much-needed rest and relaxation.

- Colouring has the power to focus the brain in much the same way meditation does. They are perfect for people who find it difficult to meditate.

- Colouring also boosts creativity and improves sleep and attention span. Colouring uses both hemispheres of the brain, hence improving our problem-solving and fine-motor skills.

- Working on such books is another way of practising mindfulness, which has therapeutic and health benefits. This helps us replace negative thoughts with positive ones.

THE IMPACT OF CLIMATE CHANGE ON HEALTH

The climate is changing. Why aren't we?

The COVID-19 pandemic changed the way we experience life in so many ways. One of the most drastic impacts was on the environment when half the world was forced to stay home, and reduce movement and travel. All those days, I woke up to a clear, blue sky instead of the smoggy, unclear one I've gotten used to in the years I've lived in Mumbai. With no vehicles on the streets and polluting industries shut, people were able to breathe probably the cleanest air of their lives. It's a pity it took a life-threatening virus to steer us to a way of life we should anyway strive for.

Our reckless and ignorant attitude towards the environment has brought us where we are today. We are all guilty of willingly choosing the things that convenience us, no matter how much it endangers others. As long as it doesn't harm us, as long as our needs are met, we're ready to turn a blind eye to the destruction we leave in our wake. I see children learning about various subjects in school and then spending more hours gaining more knowledge, but yet not enough to change their lives in a way that they can reduce pollution in their surroundings and work to reverse it.

According to the National Green Tribunal, more than 60 per cent of sewage generated by urban India is untreated and enters water bodies, such as rivers, making the water in them unfit for consumption.[1] We somehow think that whatever we throw away will be cleaned by someone else. It's an ignorant attitude, and we need to raise our children to be responsible for their own actions. Littering, even if it is a small packet of single-use plastic, doesn't do any immediate harm, but this attitude is part of the reason we are the fifth most polluted country in the world. People blame it on several things, but it's never themselves. The power to reverse ecological damage lies with the people, but we often forget the responsibilities that accompany that power.

I learnt a lot more about our impact on the environment when I took up an online course offered by Harvard University during the lockdown. I discovered just how badly we have abused our planet without realizing that we have abused ourselves in the process. Working out regularly and eating healthy can mean very little when the air we breathe is of poor quality. We are all partly responsible for that unbreathable air. By not taking care of the environment, we are endangering the lives of our children and our grandchildren. If you're as old as I am, think back to your childhood. Wasn't the environment much cleaner then? In just thirty to forty years—barely a blip when we consider the age of the Earth—we have damaged

---

[1] 'National Workshop on Redefining Urban Water Space at TERI School of Advanced Studies, Delhi', https://www.noticebard.com/workshop-redefining-urban-water-space-teri-school-advanced-studies-delhi/ (accessed on 3 August 2020).

our planet to such a grave extent that we, along with other living creatures, are all struggling to live. If just a few decades can do this, imagine how bad it will be in the next couple of decades. I shudder at the thought.

That is why I decided to include this chapter in my book. Turning a blind eye towards climate change does not make you immune to it. I hope better awareness will help you take a step towards a better life for yourself and the coming generations.

How Climate Change Affects All of Us

Climate change is the biggest global health threat of the twenty-first century. It is responsible for more heat waves, extreme weather, the spread of disease, increasing pollution and reduced productivity. In addition to direct effects such as storms, floods and fires, climate change will also contribute indirectly to decreased crop yields, overwhelmed water systems, people losing their homes and a rise in mental-health problems. Power outages in extreme weather could cripple hospitals and transportation systems. Decline in crop yields could lead to malnutrition, hunger and higher food prices. Occupational hazards, such as risk of heatstroke, especially among farmers and construction workers, will rise. Hotter days, more rain and higher humidity will produce more bacteria and viruses, which will lead to the spread of more infectious diseases. Trauma from floods, droughts, heat waves and diseases will lead to mental-health issues such as anxiety and depression.

In mid-2020, I remember how everyone around me reacted when we got the news that Cyclone Nisarga might hit Mumbai. It was something that we had no control over, which led to their instinctive reaction in such cases—panic. Such cyclones and storms will be the first of many, a result of the damage we have done. Think of yourself and the effect on your psyche when you've been in a high-risk situation that you have no control over. Now imagine that on a daily basis. That is how unpredictable life will become if we continue to pollute this beautiful planet that we inhabit.

Many people argue that we are the rightful owners of the planet. I don't agree with this, but even if we consider ourselves the caretakers of the planet, why aren't we also holding ourselves responsible for its decline? Do you see animals that have been on Earth longer than humans litter and cause active harm to it? It is time we learnt from our mistakes and strove for a better future, and finally made a change.

Hotter temperatures are causing problems ranging from respiratory and cardiac diseases to heat exhaustion and cognitive issues. Extreme weather conditions are causing direct risks to human lives by leading to the spread of various infectious diseases.

a. *The Curse of Rising CO_2*

The continued burning of fossil fuels and destruction of forests are the main factors that have fuelled the increase of carbon dioxide in our atmosphere. Excess carbon dioxide causes breathing issues. Other adverse effects include headaches, vertigo, double vision, inability to concentrate and seizures. These are just the short-term effects of breathing in this gas. Changes in bone calcium and metabolism are long-term effects.

b. Heat Waves

The increase of greenhouse gases such as carbon dioxide and methane has resulted in heat waves, where days are getting hotter. Extreme heat can lead to more droughts and hot, dry conditions can, in turn, spark off wildfires. It also affects our health in a scary way, especially of those living in urban areas. In cities, buildings, roads and other infrastructure get hot during the day, while natural surfaces remain closer to air temperatures. At night, these structures release heat slowly, which keeps cities much hotter than their surrounding areas. This is known as the urban heat island effect.

Normally, the body can cool itself through sweating. But when humidity is high, sweat will not evaporate as quickly and it could lead to a heatstroke. High humidity and increased night-time temperatures are among the main reasons of heat-related illnesses and death. Higher temperatures are also linked to an increase in cardiovascular and respiratory complications and kidney disease, and can be especially harmful to those who work outdoors.

There's enough data to back all this up, especially from people who are working on the ground in India itself. 'We find that more than 60 per cent of India has experienced significant warming during the 1951–2015 observed record. The rise in summer temperature is already more than one degree in the last 60 or so years,' said Vimal Mishra of the Water and Climate Lab at Indian Institute of Technology in Gandhinagar.[2]

We not only have to consider the immediate impact of higher temperatures but also the staggered effect it will have. For instance, heat waves caused by excess greenhouse gases can lead to drought, which could lead to lower crop yield. Food scarcity would only invite malnutrition, which can lead to a host of illnesses. People who are ill and weak are, in turn, at higher risk of being affected by heat waves. It's a vicious circle that can only be broken when we take care of our health by taking care of the environment.

c. *Ozone*

Ozone is a gas that has two functions. In the stratosphere, it absorbs harmful ultraviolet rays from the sun. But near the Earth's surface, it is a pollutant and contributes to smog. Ground-level ozone is emitted from industrial facilities and electric utilities, motor-vehicle exhaust, petrol vapours and chemical solvents. Breathing ozone can result in chest pain, throat irritation, coughing and congestion. If you are already suffering from bronchitis and asthma, it makes these conditions worse.

---

[2] 'Large parts of India have warmed, hit by frequent hot days, say climate scientists', Paradise-city.org/, 11 March 2020, https://www.paradise-city.org/large-parts-of-india-have-warmed-hit-by-frequent-hot-days-say-climate-scientists/ (accessed on 17 August 2020).

Ozone affects not just humans but plants too. It is known to cause changes in how nutrients are distributed within the plant and how they grow.

More ozone is formed in summer because there is more ultraviolent radiation from the sun then. It has been estimated that ozone mortality will be more pronounced in India and China, eastern United States, most of Europe and southern Africa.

d. More Infectious Diseases

While it's impossible to ignore the destruction that COVID-19 unleashed on our lives, we can't forget malaria, dengue, gastroenteritis, the West Nile virus, cholera and Lyme disease, which are all climate-sensitive. They are expected to worsen as climate change results in higher temperatures and more extreme weather conditions. For instance, dengue infects about forty crore people each year, especially in tropical countries such as India. According to the Intergovernmental Panel on Climate Change, the rise in temperatures, along with an increase in population, could put many more people at risk of being infected by it. The reproductive, survival and biting rates of the *Aedes aegypti* mosquito species, which carries dengue, are strongly influenced by temperature, precipitation and humidity. Mosquitoes are cold-blooded creatures and seek out warmer environments to regulate their body temperatures. The intensification of the water cycle with climate change is particularly relevant to mosquitoes' reproduction, which happens in water. If the water cycle intensifies, it means that all of its components are enhanced—so more evaporation, more precipitation and more run-off. Frequent flooding and irregular rain can also cause sudden outbreaks of dengue and malaria.

Greenhouse gases have an equal or greater relevance to the spread of infectious diseases. Rising temperatures and changing rainfall patterns have a huge impact on the way infectious diseases spread, especially through insect vectors and contaminated water. Higher emission of greenhouse gases also impacts the nutrient content in food. A higher carbon dioxide concentration reduces nutrients such as proteins, vitamin A and folate, which are already in short supply for lakhs of people around the world.

When the sea level rises due to higher temperatures, salt water intrudes upon rocks and soil. That is how it makes its way into fresh water. Crops need fresh water to grow, not salt water.

Some cities have drain pipes that carry stormwater run-off and sewage together. When the sewage system runs at full capacity, the sludge runs into local water bodies so that it doesn't back up in the system. This results in more water-borne diseases, because our drinking water comes from these local water bodies, such as lakes. We can reduce this contamination in cities by planting more vegetation and reducing the area of paved surfaces.

e. Health Disorders Caused by Fertilizers

Algal and cynobacterial blooms act like plants but produce toxins that are harmful to wildlife and humans. Warmer ocean temperatures and precipitation promote the growth of algal and cynobacterial blooms, whose main ingredient is nitrogen. The heavy use of nitro-based fertilizers to grow our food causes a range of illnesses in human beings, such as headaches, vomiting, diarrhoea, numbness and tingling.

You may be aware of a lot of things I have mentioned here. But now is the time to take action to make sure you do not contribute to these factors. We know what a healthy, clean environment can do. During the lockdown, when we were all stuck at home, nature flourished. Animals, such as deer, rhinos and elephants, who had been driven into smaller and smaller wooded areas, started coming out on the streets. People living in Jalandhar, Punjab, could see the Dhauladhar mountain range of the Himalayas, located about 200 km away, for the first time in thirty years.[3] The air quality index of Delhi, which clocks a dangerous 400 on some days, came down to 14. Instead of the haze and smog that is a constant presence in our Indian cities, people were treated to clear skies and views. The change was so remarkable that I even

---

[3] Rob Picheta, 'People in India Can See the Himalayas for the First Time in "Decades", as the Lockdown Eases Air Pollution', CNN, 9 April 2020, https://edition.cnn.com/travel/article/himalayas-visible-lockdown-india-scli-intl/index.html (accessed on 17 August 2020).

saw birds that I had not seen in more than twenty-five years of living in my house.

While governments need to bring out drastic changes in policy to go green, on an individual level there is a lot we can do too. After all, when a toxic environment can affect our health so badly, how can we not make changes to our lifestyles? We can all contribute in the simplest ways, whether it is by walking or hopping on to a bicycle instead of taking the car to places that are close to us. Not only will this result in more exercise, but it will also ensure the air we breathe is cleaner.

A clean environment is one of the vital foods of a balanced life. As we work internally and externally on making ourselves happier and our lives more fulfilled, we also have to be mindful that our existence doesn't impact the world adversely. After all, all that we do today affects our children's and grandchildren's lives in the future. I don't want my loved ones to struggle to breathe clean air because of our ignorance and mistakes. Do you?

How to Combat Climate Change

Invest in solar, wind and water energy: There are substantial health benefits of decarbonization. When governments and individuals opt for alternative sources of energy, the world can reduce its reliance on fossil fuels. While there is intermittent availability of sun and wind power, cost-effective batteries help in storage. Our family home will use solar for all our power needs from 2021.

Build better buildings: The construction and operation of buildings account for about one-third of global energy use and slightly more than one-third of global greenhouse gas emissions. Given how much electricity and energy buildings consume, carbon mitigation targeting the prevention of the worst of climate-change impact on health has to be addressed by the building sector. Several countries have started this by adopting the green building movement. It calls for more energy-efficient and environmentally friendly construction practices, which also facilitate water efficiency and waste handling. We should ensure that all roofs and balconies, even our building compounds, have plenty of plants. Surrounding ourselves with greenery will do wonders for our health.

Reduce the use of air conditioners: Turning on the air conditioner is the fastest way to beat the heat. But it causes a vicious cycle, where using the appliance itself contributes to an increase in heat waves. More demand for air conditioning increases the need for more power. That, in turn, means more emissions and even hotter temperatures. Air-conditioning units funnel heat outside, exacerbating the urban heat island effect. By keeping them on for less time and relying on fans to ease the heat, we will all be doing our bit to stem the rapid increase of climate change.

Reduce over-reliance on fossil fuels: Globally, fossil fuels, including coal and natural gas, dominate the production of electricity. Burning of these fossil fuels releases a lot of pollutants in the environment. Around 10 lakh Indians die every year from air pollution.[4] It even pollutes the food we eat. Fish have been seen to have elevated levels of mercury as a result of human use of coal. Globally, we

---

[4] 'Air Pollution Kills 10 Lakh Indians Every Year: Study', *The Hindu*, 19 February 2017, https://www.thehindu.com/sci-tech/energy-and-environment/two-indians-die-every-minute-due-to-air-pollution-study/article17328922.ece (accessed on 17 August 2020).

consume the equivalent of more than 11 billion tonnes of oil from fossil fuels every year. Crude oil reserves are vanishing at a rate of more than 4 billion tonnes a year, so if we carry on as we are, our known oil deposits could run out in just around fifty-three years.[5]

Go vegan: Agriculture accounts for about a quarter of greenhouse gas emissions. Livestock rearing for human consumption contributes to global warming through the methane that animals produce, but also via deforestation to expand their pastures. If land is used more effectively, it can store more of the carbon emitted by humans. So the best way we can all contribute to a better world is by consuming a plant-based diet. Food processing, storage and distribution accounts for 20–30 per cent of greenhouse gas emissions.[6]

Waste less food: The IPCC has estimated that greenhouse emissions associated with food loss and waste—from fields to the kitchen bin—is as high as 8–10 per cent of all global emissions.[7] The carbon footprint of all the food we throw

---

5   'When Fossil Fuels Run Out, What Then?', MAHB, May 2019, https://mahb.stanford.edu/library-item/fossil-fuels-run/ (accessed on 17 August 2020).

6   'Agriculture and Food Production Contribute Up to 29 Percent of Global Greenhouse Gas Emissions According to Comprehensive Research Papers', CCAFS, 31 October 2012, https://ccafs.cgiar.org/news/press-releases/agriculture-and-food-production-contribute-29-percent-global-greenhouse-gas#.Xyvoa4gzbIU (accessed on 17 August 2020).

7   'A New Diet to Combat the Climate Crisis', Iberdrola, https://www.iberdrola.com/environment/food-waste#:~:text=FOOD%20WASTE%20AND%20THE%20CLIMATE%20CRISIS%3A%20

away is 4.4 billion metric tonnes of carbon dioxide.[8] Also, wasted food uses 45 trillion gallons of water, which is 25 per cent of all the water used for agriculture globally.[9] By recycling food and ensuring that all excess is consumed by those less fortunate, we can reduce the rate at which climate change occurs.

I strongly believe that once our mindset changes, everything else will follow. In school and college, we're taught about finance, science and history, yet spreading knowledge about the environment is overlooked and treated as less significant. We are raising our children to be intelligent enough to hold top rankings in prestigious universities around the world but ignorant of how the world is inhabited, polluted and taken for granted. For every action, there is an equal and opposite reaction. It's time we inculcate respect for the planet in our lives rather than just our test papers and studies, and understand that every negative action of ours has an equal or more drastic effect on our planet. Climate change is more real than ever now. It is time to act.

THE%20IPCC%20REPORT&text=These%20data%20come%20from%20the,in%20the%20period%202010%2D2016.

[8] 'Food Wastage Footprint & Climate Change', Food and Agriculture Organization of the United Nations, http://www.fao.org/3/a-bb144e.pdf (accessed on 17 August 2020).

[9] John Hawthorne, '5 ways food waste is destroying our beautiful planet', *New Food*, 9 August 2017, https://www.newfoodmagazine.com/article/43551/five-ways-food-waste-environment/#:~:text=All%20told%2C%20if%20the%20 1.3,freshwater%20is%20used%20for%20agriculture (accessed on 17 August 2020).

CONCLUSION

Say it with me: I am strong. I am smart. I am capable.
I am able. I am valid.

My laptop is facing my open balcony; I can hear birds chirping; and the peepul tree is swaying in the summer breeze as I type these words. As I sit down to write my final chapter, I think of the coronavirus pandemic and how it has affected our world, but only one word comes to my mind if I need to sum it all up—survival. It's been the driving factor behind the strength of the human race—adaptability and the ability to strive for a brighter day. Of course, the world has suffered terrible losses, but it's also shown that no matter the scale of the problem, humans have the capability to come together to find a solution. It is this hope, with the right choices and the right balance, that makes life beautiful.

Most people lived a completely different life during the lockdown. It made them spend more time with their family, have a chance to reflect on different aspects of their situation, connect with people and pitch in to share housework. On a personal level too, it encouraged people to look inwards, understand their needs and take up new things to learn in their free time.

Self-discipline is a core aspect of remote work. But, more importantly, it is a core aspect of growth too. Self-discipline begins with your habits. The lockdown gave us an opportunity to form new habits and kill old ones. Little to no travel time definitely made way for more time to work out, meditate, eat fresh and work. Most importantly, I hope it gave you time to pause, to take a step back and observe your own life. That's something that is so necessary for us all to do, regardless of the situation. Knowing yourself and knowing what you need is so essential to achieving balance in your life. If you can't evaluate which part of the circle of life needs more attention than the other, how will you be able to work towards that balance? So every time you feel bogged down, tired or demotivated, ask yourself what you would like to stop doing. What would you like to do more?

Change now. Begin now.

The strength of human dedication and determination is immense. If we individually and collectively put our minds to a problem, nothing can stop us from solving it.

This is the life I have been living for a long time now. I'm thankful that by focusing on the different aspects of my life, I have been able to find happiness, fulfilment and balance. When we slow down, we realize that the only things that matter in life are family, friends, love, health, financial stability and creative output. That is what the balance of life is all about. It's this magic of balance that this book is about. And, in many ways, the pandemic brought us all closer—it made us all stop and think about our actions and intentions, and what needs to change in the future. When entire societies and countries bowed down to the coronavirus, we realized how valuable certain freedoms are and how none of it should be taken for granted.

I hope one of the most important lessons you can take away from this book is the concept of bio-individuality. As you've learnt, it is a concept that stresses on the fact that the issues we all face are personalized, and thus the solutions have to be customized too. What works for someone else—whether it is in career, relationships, fitness or health—may not work for you. To illustrate it simply, if you aren't fond of bananas, the best banana bread in the world—even if it is made by the best chefs in the world—won't be appealing to you. You will always choose what you like.

Similarly, no matter what advice anyone gives you on how you should conduct your financial matters, career choices, relationship issues or fitness goals, it may not suit you. In every instance, you need something that works for you. I could write five more books on the importance of balance in life, but if you don't seek that balance within yourself, you will not find it. I cannot promise you that by reading this book you will have achieved balance overnight, but what I can promise you is that if you start looking at life in the way that this book talks about—by not overdoing, nor underdoing, but just doing, by just striking that equilibrium—you will feel more content than ever.

It's important to remember to be at peace and strive for calm and happiness. In your quest to improve your life, do not become obsessed with achieving your dream body or finding your dream career, partner and life. Just do your best with earnestness and sincerity. The results and the balance will follow.

Once you start understanding the role balance plays in every endeavour, you'll realize that this world has always strived and moved forward because of it. Every single action can be overdone or underdone. It is equilibrium that leads to beauty, perfection and contentment.

Most people aim for the stars, and forget that between the sea and the stars, lies the earth. While aiming for the stars, we forget to keep our feet on the ground—and that is why we lose this balance. So be in the moment, even if you're looking to the future. If the past takes up too much space in your mind, let it go and embrace the beauty of life. Let it sweep you off your feet. Let your innocence flow back into you. When every facet of your life is in balance, you will flourish and be in a state of nirvana with the peace and happiness that you desire.

I hope this books helps you get closer to balancing your life. I'd love to hear from you and how you are using tips from this book. You can message me on Instagram @deannepanday as well as write to me at deannepanday@gmail.com or on www.deannepanday.com. Till then, happy reading and wishing you the best that life has to offer.

ACKNOWLEDGEMENTS

Thank you to my lifelong friends—my children Alanna and Ahaan. Never forget that I love you. For all the things my hands have held, you two are the best by far. You are the gifts for everything I did right in my life.

To my husband Chikki—without you, I wouldn't have learnt how to turn pain into power. Thank you for being the best cook I have ever known and for being my best friend.

I am thankful for my puppy, Peach, for coming into our lives just before Sukhi, our fifteen-year-old doggie, left us. Peach, you are happiness. And Cappucino, my kitty, thank you for teaching us patience.

A big thank you to Nihal Ketan Ruparel and Haider Khan, who shot the photographs for the front and the back covers, respectively. They wouldn't have turned out as beautifully without Rocky Star styling me for the front cover and Nandita Mahtani styling me for the back cover.

Parita, I can't forget all the hours we sat together, day in and day out, working on this book together. Thank you for this wonder you helped me create.

Thank you, Milee and Roshini, for all your support and help.

I wouldn't be the same person without the knowledge and encouragement I have received from my school, the Institute of Integrative Nutrition. I will always try to pass on all I have learnt and create a ripple effect of goodness, wellness and health.